3 week
649.33
SMA

Accession no.
01086904

D0625556

R02697

wARR

THE NATIONAL CHILDBIRTH TRUST
Book of Breastfeeding

THE NATIONAL
CHILDBIRTH TRUST

Book of
Breastfeeding

Practical solutions to your day-to-day problems

MARY SMALE

VERMILION
LONDON

4339501003098442772601 2

1 3 5 7 9 10 8 6 4 2

Text copyright © NCT Trading Ltd and Mary Smale 1992, 1999
Illustrations © Random House Group Ltd 1999

The right of Mary Smale and The National Childbirth Trust to be
identified as the authors of this book has been asserted by them in
accordance with the Copyright, Designs and Patents Act 1988.

All rights reserved. No part of the publication may be reproduced,
stored in a retrieval system, or transmitted in any form or by any
means, electronic, mechanical, photocopying, recording or otherwise, without the prior permission of the copyright owners.

First published in the United Kingdom in 1992 by Vermilion
This new edition published in the United Kingdom in 1999 by Vermilion
an imprint of Ebury Press
Random House
20 Vauxhall Bridge Road
London SW1V 2SA

Random House Australia (Pty) Limited
20 Alfred Street, Milsons Point, Sydney
New South Wales 2061, Australia

Random House New Zealand Limited
18 Poland Road, Glenfield
Auckland 10, New Zealand

Random House (Pty) Limited
Endulini, 5A Jubilee Road,
Parktown 2193, South Africa

Random House Group Ltd Reg. No. 954009
www.randomhouse.co.uk

A CIP catalogue record for this book
is available from the British Library

ISBN 0 09 182569 5

Printed and bound in by Biddles of Guildford

Contents

Preface

The author would like to thank the Breastfeeding Promotion Group of the National Childbirth Trust for thinking this book was a good idea, and believing I could write it, Suzanne Dobson for calm support throughout the venture, and the following people for detailed help – Dora Henschel, Shirleyanne Seel, Deborah Young, Anne Buckley, Alison Spiro, Patricia Donnithorne, Gill Mitchell and Naomi Beckles-Wilson. Above all, many thanks to Pat Lawrence to whom I 'drip-fed' the book, chapter by chapter as it was being written, for valued and constructive feedback.

In one way the book is for my own daughters although they pointed out that, having overheard so much 'breastfeeding talk', they might be the last ones to need it. They are one reason why all the babies in this book are 'she's'. It was they who taught me what to do and how much it meant to do it, and then put up with me being on the phone while I tried to help other mothers. The book would also have been impossible without the encouragement and support of my husband who numbers expert breakfast-making among his many domestic skills. This habit began as a direct result of breastfeeding, while I did the morning feeds, and has carried on for 18 years because he is more awake at 7 o'clock than I am, and is a simple example of the way that life with a baby can change people. Thanks to Hilary English for reading this 1999 edition as it was brought up to date and also for supplying line drawings about how a baby can best approach feeding. Thanks also to Rosemary Dodds, Caroline Harris, Wendy Jones and Alison Watts for detailed help. Any errors, as before, are the responsibility of the author.

Introduction

This book is for:

- parents who are thinking about breastfeeding for the first time. Some will bring great enthusiasm for a natural process, but may still find it helpful to know how breastfeeding works.
- parents coming with a good deal of wariness, having listened to stories of failing milk supplies or sore nipples. It need not be like that. Most mothers can feed their own babies with the right help.
- mothers who have tried breastfeeding and found there were problems and want to get it right for themselves this time.

This book grew from many people's experiences – from over 30 years of information pooled by hundreds of National Childbirth Trust breastfeeding counsellors as they listened to mothers and shared their concerns; from reading about the research on breastfeeding, and from the letters of many mothers who responded to a call for their own stories. It is their words that are printed in speech marks here. They wrote about breastfeeding and what it meant to them. Everyone who replied has raised points which are important to others. One of the questions I asked mothers who had breastfed was 'What would you have wanted to see in such a book?' A few reminded me that many mothers find no real problems in breastfeeding and cannot see the need for books or leaflets. Perhaps they were very lucky in the help they received, or particularly determined. Others wanted to pass on messages to the next group of mothers. For example, it helps to remember that every baby, and so every breastfeeding experience, is different.

It was also hoped that the book might be 'a plain down-to-earth' book as 'most pregnant women have no idea what is really involved.' Most people have met someone who has found breastfeeding difficult, and regrets this very much. So one mother felt it was important to give:

'Realistic information about how many mothers give up breastfeeding and why, so that would-be breast-feeders know what to expect and don't feel total failures when things start to go wrong. Unless women are aware of their problems, they will assume that they are unique in suffering them and will give up, especially as the problems are experienced at an emotionally vulnerable time.'

Some offered practical tips; some were concerned about social attitudes to breasts themselves, causing problems for mothers trying to breastfeed outside the home. They made suggestions for ways in which women might respond unapologetically for making the choice they have.

Feeding a baby is a process with a great deal of meaning and many women remember both trauma and delights years later, and are able to recall the details vividly: 'some of my feelings of guilt, regret and confusion remain very much with me two years after my daughter's birth.'

But not everyone has a sad tale to tell. Some were mixed, with triumphs after previous dismay, and disappointing starts leading to delight: 'I regard it now as a real achievement and one of the most rewarding experiences of my life. When I see other babies being breastfed I feel very emotional.' Others were happy experiences: 'most of the 13 months have been blissfully hassle-free'.

The mother who wrote that did have some problems early on, but they faded for her in the light of the total experience.

This book inevitably spends time on problems – but please remember that you won't get all of them. There are many women who feed for months entirely trouble free. It may help to remember that bottle-feeding is not without its problems, or mothers would not change brands so often. It is unrealistic to expect life, particularly with a baby, always to be simple.

Breastfeeding in the third millennium

This is an exciting time for anyone involved with breastfeeding. The World Health Organisation and UNICEF have made breast-feeding an important part of campaigns for child health; all over the world the Baby Friendly Initiative is setting research-based standards for hospitals which increase the likelihood that the care women and babies receive there will make breastfeeding possible. The first hospital in Britain to become 'Baby Friendly' was shown in 1995 to be working in line with ten simple steps which allow women to breastfeed more easily. Now there are over twenty such hospitals in the country, and most hospitals have begun to think very carefully about the infant feeding poli-cies and practices they have in place, making them available to mothers to explain how newer ideas are based on good research and knowledge. The Initiative is spreading to Community Trusts as well. There is encouragement for councils as well as shops and restaurants, to protect mothers from difficulties in breastfeeding away from home, putting forward a more positive image of breastfeeding as an everyday activity.

Research is continually exploring how breastfeeding works, how breastmilk is different from cow's milk formula – 'babymilk', and how best to help breastfeeding mothers. A good deal more is now known than 20 years ago, and policies in hos-pitals are changing in the light of these findings. A simple exam-ple is that most hospitals now encourage mothers to feed whenever the baby is hungry rather than wait for a set time, because it is now understood how unhelpful rigid timings are. Research has confirmed that it is best to follow the baby's needs.

The suggestions in this book may come from research – for example into what does and does not help women with inverted nipples, from knowledge – for example an understanding of how babies attach themselves to their mothers' breasts, or from the experience of women. All these suggestion are likely to change as more is understood, old ideas are abandoned and new methods are tried; while we have tried to be as up-to-date as we can, it always helps to talk about any concern you have to someone with a good understanding and current information.

We know that having someone consistent to offer good support and information is very important. Sadly we also know that it is breastfeeding which sometimes causes the most dissatisfaction for first-time mothers. Currently around two-thirds of women begin breastfeeding in the UK, but by four months fewer than one-third are still offering breastmilk at all, a very small increase on the figures of five years ago. Women stop most in the first two weeks, which are times of great change in their lives and in the breastfeeding journey. The two main reasons which mothers give for stopping feeding their babies breastmilk in the first few weeks after birth are a sense of not having enough milk and uncomfortably sore nipples.

Just as with learning any other set of skills, there is often some trepidation about your capacity to do it, fear about looking silly, getting it all wrong, failing, or even not being able to stop. We hope that this down-to-earth book will help you to conquer these worries and that it will teach you more about breastfeeding. Many voluntary organisations and knowledgeable health professionals provide help for women to continue breastfeeding as long as they want. There are no 'silly' questions for such people, so do try to find help rather than put up with difficulties at any stage. For more details of how to find an NCT breastfeeding counsellor see page 192.

Finally, an asterisk (*) occuring in the text means that a corresponding reference can be found on pages 194-195.

CHAPTER ONE

Decisions – do I want to do this?

'I was determined to breastfeed because it seemed to involve less work for me than bottle-feeding whilst giving the baby the ideal food for baby humans.'

You can only start with how you already feel. Few women decide about breastmilk or formula without giving it some thought during pregnancy, but a great deal of the evidence for your decision may have been gathered long ago. Even if you have long since decided that breastfeeding is for you, you may find this section useful in reinforcing your decision and in thinking about the reality of nurturing a baby. If you are not so sure, it would not be surprising. We do not have as many big families in which to watch breastfeeding, which is often conducted in a private setting. Many mothers' own parents were of a bottle-feeding generation, or found breastfeeding was made very difficult for them by the way it was supposed to be done 20 or 30 years ago.

Teaching in schools about this subject is still fairly rare, and although most people know that 'breast is best' for the baby, and might be able to give a few reasons, until the last few years many people had not seen a breastfeeding mother at close quarters or had the chance to ask her questions.

'When I was pregnant I felt I had visible proof that I was a woman, and delighted with the slight increase in my bust measurement . . . I did enjoy having real curves, however briefly.'

Your expectations of feeding will depend on how you see yourself (including your own feelings about your breasts), your experience of other mothers, including your own, what else is going on in your life when you become pregnant, whether you have breastfed or not before, and the stories you have heard, some of them so long ago that you have forgotten. You may have picked up very early from seeing a mother and baby how good it can feel – and not realised that this may not be an *instant* feeling, but that it grows with time and practice. Some people really look forward to learning to breastfeed and find it relaxing, others see it as a worrying challenge.

Outside influences

When deciding what is best for you and your baby, it does seem a good idea to make sure you have really chosen and not just automatically plumped for an option. There are, however, many influences which can affect your decision.

Your partner

Your partner may well have expectations. Sometimes these can be very different from yours and that can be rather a surprise. What if it is your partner who is enthusiastic and you are not sure? It is a good idea to do your thinking together. Whichever way you choose, feeding will be a main preoccupation for both of you once the baby arrives. If someone else is going to care for you after the birth as you mother your baby, it is a good idea to see what they are expecting, and what they can offer you. If they differ from you in what they think about how to feed, it is better to find out and talk about it before the baby is born.

Your family

It may be that the message in your family is that they view breastfeeding as simply being rude. You may need to decide whether to accept that or decide for yourself, and if you opt for breastfeeding, to think about how to cope with family reactions. Stories in the family – and silences – about certain topics are very powerful ways of telling us about things that matter a lot. If a family never talked about '*that* kind of thing' this is quite a strong message. Or while it is known that breastmilk is best your family might think that it should only happen in the bedroom or bathroom. Their attitude may change as they see a baby doing well on breastmilk and realise how invisible breastfeeding can be. But you will need to think about what you might do if this is your family's attitude.

Your friends

You may be the first one of your circle to be having a baby, or you may have lots of friends who have already got children. What do they do and think? Ask around, and you will find out how different everyone is. Of course, they will also have been influenced by their family and friends, and each one will have a personal outlook as well. It may help to try to understand where they got their ideas. You may find you are isolated in what you want to do: it can be hard being the only breastfeeding mother, or the only one who doesn't stop after three weeks. You might need to go outside your group to find support in your breast-feeding, as well as keeping in touch with them for friendship.

Yourself

Health workers are right to tell you that breastmilk is best for the baby but it may be hard for you to express your concerns about messiness or inconvenience. You may have strong feelings.

'For a mother who wanted to do everything "right" or "proper", it was conflicting that I felt so strongly against breastfeeding even at this early stage of pregnancy . . . posters advocating "breast is best" seemed always to stare at me . . . breastfeeding was also a personal invasion of my privacy, not an invasion by my daughter or indeed my husband, but by the rest of the world. I knew that I was going to find it embarrassing and humiliating feeding in front of others and that it was realistic to believe that somewhere private and comfortable without interruptions cannot

always be found. Perhaps I am prudish, but in a society where males gloat on women's breasts, I found it hard to make the distinction between this and their proper human function – to feed babies.'

Try to find someone who is willing to listen to any concerns and try to keep an open mind unless you are adamant about bottle-feeding, and see how you find breastfeeding. People have been known to be converted to it on the delivery table when they met their baby for the first time. It is usually seen as being easy to change to bottle-feeding and quite impossible to change to breastfeeding. In fact, it is not always totally simple to change to bottle-feeding – the baby may not like teats, and it cannot be done too fast, or you will lend up feeling very uncomfortable – but it is possible to move from bottle-feeding to breastfeeding. Some mothers have made the change after a few days of bottle-feeding, perhaps when their milk came in on about the third day after the birth, and they saw other mothers enjoying it.

Writing things down

If you are having difficulty in deciding what you want, try listing the main points at issue. Perhaps you could ask yourself:

- What are the main things I want from the way I will feed?
- What do I want for myself? for the baby? for others?
- What do I already know?
- What else do I need to know?

You and your partner or the person most likely to be around to help you initially might also find it useful to look at the following questions. You could answer the questions privately and then tell each other what you wrote and talk about any surprises you got – maybe finding some similar answers and some different ones. These may help you to identify what more you need to know. Your partner may wish to share in reading this book or something shorter, like the leaflet, 'Feeding your Baby' available from the National Childbirth Trust's Maternity Sales (see page 197 for address) or free from any Tesco store with a pharmacy.

- What feelings do you get when you think about breast-feeding?
- What kind of experience of seeing it have you had?
- What have people told you about it which encourages you?
- What are you looking forward to about it?
- What things worry you?
- Do you see it as something that happens easily, or is it sometimes difficult, or nearly always a big problem?

You could go on to write down your hopes, and to try to find out why you have chosen a particular direction by asking 'why do I believe this?' You might come up with such statements as 'it is natural', and 'I want to do the best for the baby', and you will no doubt come up with other reasons too. You could also move on to the worries that you have about breastfeeding and where you feel you might have come from. It would be interesting to test your gloomy and hopeful feelings against the information in this book, and against real life once you have your baby.

It is useful to spend time talking about your ideas with the people who are going to be your main sources of support after the baby is born, whether they are your parents, your partner or friends. It probably does not matter if you do not agree, as long as you can understand how each other feels. You may end up with a lot of questions to ask. Getting information about breastfeeding is quite easy. There is a lot of material about, but finding out which is the true picture and the one which will suit you may not be quite so simple.

The second time around, or the third, or the fourth, or . . .

One mother who found feeding her first baby so difficult that she ended up bottle-feeding, described feeding her second baby: 'I put my second son straight to the breast after his birth and he sucked immediately. We never looked back, and I fed him until he was 10 months.'

If you have tried breastfeeding before and it did not go well for you, the person who was helping may have felt very sad for you and also helpless. Whoever was supporting you as a new mother may feel it is not a good idea even to try again, or hope that this time it will come right, as if breastfeeding was a matter of 'luck'. Before making another attempt, it can be useful to talk to someone who will listen carefully to you if there are still parts of the feeding experience of a previous baby which sadden or puzzle you. Not only can you clear up some facts, and perhaps find an explanation for what happened, but also it may help you to come to terms with how feeding went. Breastfeeding counsellors are trained to use counselling skills to help women to do this, and offer a confidential service. If you want to speak to one, try looking up National Childbirth Trust in the phone book or get in touch with the headquarters number at the back of this book to find your nearest breastfeeding counsellor's phone number.

'I assumed it would be a piece of cake as it was the "natural" way to do things . . . by the time I was deemed well enough to go home I thoroughly disliked this scrap of humanity and I particularly disliked breastfeeding. It was painful, awkward and I found it totally repulsive.'

Even if you found that you did not like the sensations of breastfeeding and have mixed feelings about attempting again, it can help to talk about this, to help you to decide what is right for you. No one should try to persuade you to breastfeed if you did not like it, but you may find it helpful to use someone else as a sounding board while you put your finger on what it was that you did not like. If it was uncomfortable, then information about ways to position the baby comfortably at the breast should help. If you found it messy, there may be useful tips, and if there was something about it which really put you off, then it can help to acknowledge this.

Information

Getting reliable information about breastfeeding is an important part of preparation. You can obviously begin by talking to mothers who are currently feeding in various ways, as well as to your own family and friends. As the pregnancy progresses you should also meet midwives, including perhaps one who will care for you during at least the first ten days after the birth when you come home. It is good to find out real answers and not rely on the myths that often put people off breastfeeding.

Antenatal classes

Antenatal classes are a good place to focus on feeding as well as birth preparation: 'I was very naive about motherhood, but I was fairly certain I wanted to breastfeed. By the time I'd been churned through NHS classes I was absolutely convinced.' National Health classes are usually available, held in clinics and hospitals, during the day and in the evenings and partners can attend as well. These are run by midwives or health visitors. Their knowledge of local breastfeeding practices will be useful, and as midwives sometimes 'rotate' from antenatal to postnatal care, you may even see some familiar faces from your classes after the birth. You may meet 'your' health visitor too, who will be involved in the care of your baby and young child right up to school age, taking over from the midwife. Sometimes parents from a previous class are invited back to talk to members about the reality of life with a new baby. You may also see a video or two about feeding.

Films, videos and tapes

Some of the material you come across may well be directly or indirectly funded by formula manufacturers. So bear in mind that in the long run they may be interested in your loyalty to a particular brand of formula milk. Their information may well be correct but they can subtly sow the seeds of distrust in breastfeeding. Talk to the health professional involved if you are wondering about this.

Visual images give a useful opportunity to look out for ways in which bottle-feeding and breastfeeding have very different techniques for mothers. One involves learning about measuring and sterilising. The other mainly concentrates on the very different skill of positioning the baby on the breast without any need to worry about getting the contents of the breasts right at all.

'We learned at the NCT breastfeeding class that it didn't always turn out to be straightforward, but like everybody else we thought that wouldn't be us.'

National Childbirth Trust classes

The National Childbirth Trust also runs antenatal classes for parents, usually with small numbers, as they are generally in someone's house, sometimes providing 'mothers only' groups. During a course of classes, it is likely that you would meet a breastfeeding counsellor or antenatal teacher who explores with the group what the parents feel about feeding and gives basic information about how to begin breastfeeding. She will also help you to think about coping with some possible problems, and most important of all perhaps, give you her phone number and those of other local breastfeeding counsellors to contact should you want to speak to someone. (She would love to hear if all is well too; anyone can consult a breastfeeding counsellor before or after birth.) Parents of breastfed babies will often return during one of the later classes to talk about their birth and early breastfeeding experiences, answer questions, and sometimes – if the baby is cooperative – feed the baby.

In any classes you will be able to meet other people in the same situation as you and share ideas about labour, birth and parenting as well as getting information from health professionals or NCT trained antenatal teachers and breastfeeding counsellors. Many mothers and fathers make lasting friendships at such gatherings. For second-time parents with toddlers and jobs, it is perhaps the only time to focus on the new arrival, and to try to think about the experience they would like *this* time.

Books, leaflets and magazines

It can help to read about how breastfeeding works, partly so that you can understand how it may be that other women's experiences of 'not enough milk' or 'sore nipples' were not just matters of chance but happened for reasons, and might have been avoided or helped. Mother and baby magazines can also be a good source of information and you can see what kind of things mothers write in about.

Some common questions

Q *Will it take me longer to get back to normal if I breastfeed?*
A It depends what you mean by normal of course. If you are thinking of being able to get out for an evening or go to the nearest town on your own for a while, it may be possible quite soon to leave the baby and some breastmilk, although you may find you are not able to forget her as easily as you might expect. You may find yourself getting uncomfortable with full breasts and needing to express some milk. So you may find it better to take the baby to do this for you while you are away from home.

One of the ways in which breastfeeding is often said to be better than bottle-feeding is that women 'get their figures back more quickly'. This may mean that you will get your waist back more quickly as the womb shrinks more rapidly if you breastfeed. (You can sometimes actually feel that happening.) Of course, it is likely that your breasts will be bigger as you breastfeed, especially initially, and this can feel like a good thing or an embarrassment. You put on around half a stone during pregnancy ready for feeding, and it seems that this is easier to move if you use it up in the way for which it was designed. This may not happen right away, and some women find they do not lose this weight until after they have finished feeding. Most breastfeeding mothers have a very healthy appetite though, and find they can eat fairly well without gaining too much weight.

Q *Isn't formula milk just as good nowadays?*
A Manufacturers of breastmilk substitute do a great deal of research so that their recipe is as accurate a chemical imitation of breastmilk as possible, using cow's milk and other ingredients, like soya or coconut. By adding and subtracting various carbohydrates, fats, proteins, vitamins and minerals, they arrive at a safe product. New, small alterations are being made all the time as research on breastmilk shows the importance of particular proteins and so on. It seems very unlikely, however, that infant formula will ever accurately reproduce the living part of breast-

milk which contains the antibodies against diseases that you have encountered, the immunoglobulins which protect the baby against some allergic conditions, or the special additive which stops bacteria from being able to use the iron in your baby. The manufacturers are working on this but the difficulties, in terms of the cost alone, make it very unlikely that formula will ever completely imitate breastmilk. The adaptability of breastmilk to the individual baby is not something which can be easily imitated by a packet, which is why a mother with a thirsty bottle-fed baby needs to be aware she may need to give water. Breastmilk relies on a more subtle system and as long as the mother follows the baby's wishes, the baby's needs can be met without any intervention.

Most parents know that breastfeeding is healthier for their baby, but they may not know the details. Breastmilk is not just like an immunisation providing protection against diseases the mother meets but has various ways of safeguarding the baby against infection and allergies and priming the baby's own defences. There is now more research about this area than ever before. Basically the greater the proportion of breastmilk you can give the better. For example, in Britain a bottle-fed baby is five times more likely to be admitted to hospital with the effects of stomach bugs.* Babies fed exclusively on breastmilk get half the number of middle ear infections on average compared with those who also get formula.** Statistics such as these – and your health professionals can tell you more if you feel you need to know – are cited here not to make you feel anxious but to be useful to you when other people suggest that breastfeeding is too much like hard work or not worthwhile.

Q *Are there any health benefits for me?*
A Quite a few: a couple of quick examples are that there is less breast cancer before the menopause the longer you breastfeed and a lower chance of hip fractures because of osteoporosis later on.***

Q *If I breastfeed should I buy bottles and things?*
A If you are intending to return to work or leave the baby occasionally with a bottle of your own milk while you go out, or your

partner wants to be able to feed the baby sometimes by bottle, then you may want to look around at what is available while you are comparatively free to shop in peace. As you will read later in the book, babies can all too quickly come to prefer bottle-feeding, so if you know you will be needing to use a bottle at some stage, experience suggests it is a good idea to wait until you have both felt quite comfortable with breastfeeding for a couple of weeks before offering a teat to your baby. On the other hand, it is probably a good idea not to wait until later than six weeks or so after birth. If you are not intending to use bottles, you may still have people suggest it is wise to have one or two 'just in case'. Babies can be fed from a sterilised spoon or a little cup in an emergency. There is certainly no need to buy a sterilising kit; all you need is a good quality plastic container which will hold enough water to cover any bottles, a bottle brush and sterilising liquid or tablets which are available from any chemist.

Q *Will I be able to find the time to breastfeed?*
A This can be a real worry, especially for mothers who already have one or more children. Breastfeeding does take a while to learn, and babies will have periods when they are feeding a lot, but once it is running smoothly, mothers who enjoy it find it is actually far less trouble than bottle-feeding. It may be that you have heard the stories of mothers who gave up breastfeeding because the baby was feeding 'all the time'. There is usually an explanation for this, and feeds should not be taking hours and hours and continually running into one another. It is more likely that something needs putting right. Breastfeeding is not always like that. When babies are young they often feed on and off all evening, and it is useful to know that this is normal and will pass. They may also have brief periods of especially frequent feeding from time to time (see p. 81–2). We are very used in our world now to being able to shop whenever we want or to make television programmes wait on video till we are ready to watch them. You may need to give yourself time to get used to a less predictable lifestyle than the one you may be used to. Feeding is just one part of that – bottle feeding is usually now done on demand too. It can feel strange to have to fit in with a small baby, but as you read this book it may become clearer how rational this way

of feeding is. Feeds do get shorter and usually a more obvious pattern in their spacing emerges as time goes on as well.

Q *Will my baby sleep longer and more regularly if I bottle-feed?*
A The unpredictable nature of breastfeeding – what is called 'demand' feeding – can be worrying, perhaps mainly for the other people around a mother, who often pass on their concern to her. However, as formula is now chemically closer to breast-milk and so digested quite quickly, demand feeding is acceptable for bottle-fed babies, too.

On the whole, breastfed babies do sleep through the night a few weeks later than bottle-fed ones, but it is usually easier to settle them back to sleep with a quick feed and a cuddle, rather than having to wake up enough to warm a bottle.

Q *Do I have to eat special foods and avoid things I like?*
A Whatever you eat will turn into breastmilk. If your diet is not quite right in some way, your milk-making cells will just use your own body stores of whatever is missing to supply the quite small amounts required for the baby. A wide range of foods, with plenty of fresh fruit and vegetables, will provide you and the baby with energy and growth. Cows don't drink milk, and nor do you need to unless you like it. There is no problem for vegetarians who want to breastfeed, although vegans who eat no animal products at all may need to take some supplementary vitamin B12. Your own societies, or community dietician, can help. Some mothers find their babies react badly to something they have eaten, so they stop eating it for about a week, before trying again.

Q *Can I do it?*
A With good knowledge and support, most women can breast-feed. There are a very few special health problems which may make it impossible or difficult to breastfeed, mainly because of the treatments needed, and you need to speak to those caring for you if this is so. Sometimes, alternative drugs which are less likely to upset the baby may be possible. An NCT breastfeeding counsellor will be able to find out more for you about drugs you are taking.

Q *Am I the type?*
A You do not have to be a particular sort of person to be able to breastfeed. You may find it helpful to find out more about breastfeeding and speak to a number of women who have done it before you decide about it. No one is quite the same after a baby, and you can surprise yourself. If you thought you were too tidy, too career-minded, too modern or too anything else, you might think quite differently after the arrival of your baby. It is quite possible to do more than one job at once, and breastfeeding can be combined with all kinds of things like reading, talking, making toast, playing with a toddler or eating a meal, or doing a part- or full-time job.

Q *Am I too old?*
A You may have been surprised if you are over the age of 30 to find that you are regarded as 'elderly'. In the past, some problems experienced by older mothers were blamed on this fact alone, but most mothers who decide to have a baby after a longish period in a career are able to feed them as well as make them.

Q *Is there any point in starting to breastfeed if I am going back to work?*
A Research suggests that breastmilk for at least the first 13 weeks gives benefit to babies in protecting them from tummy bugs and chest infections. There are all kinds of other reasons, too, why you may feel that you want to breastfeed, even if only for a few weeks. Many women do combine a career and breastfeeding, even if it is partial, and find it a good way to feel really in touch with their babies.

Q *My nipples don't look like other women's.*
A If you have flat nipples or inverted ones, which turn in when you touch them, it is still usually possible to breastfeed. A large research project has found that preparations like wearing special breastshells or rolling the nipple antenatally made no difference to women with inverted nipples.* It may be reassuring to know that many nipples which do not stand out before pregnancy

often begin to do so as the baby starts to feed. In any case, as you will see later, the baby is not going to pull on your nipple like she would a teat, but is going to take in quite a lot of your breast tissue as well (see Chapter 2).

Q *Do I have to do things beforehand to get ready?*
A Preparing for breastfeeding used to be a horrendous ritual. There was the nailbrush, harsh towel and expressing of colostrum. Now we know that these are unhelpful and were only thought necessary because at the time it was felt that nipples must need toughening up. Now the usual advice is that while you are pregnant, you should simply avoid using any scented products, including soap, on your nipples. This avoids drying out the skin which will be kept supple by secretions from the little bumps around the edge of the areola – the circle of darker skin which lies around the nipple.

Preparation

If you are bottle-feeding you need to buy all kinds of equipment and then you can feel ready, but with breastfeeding, you just need to know that your own body is doing the work of getting ready without you needing to do anything.

While you are pregnant, you are, of course, already feeding the baby through the umbilical cord. You are probably more aware than ever before of the need for care about what you eat but without having to worry about how much or how often the baby is to be fed. Meanwhile, your breasts are preparing for the next stage of the baby's dependence on you for food. They are becoming compact milk factories, ready to operate after the birth. Whether your breasts are large, small, pointed, or long, this process happens to almost 100 per cent of all mothers. While you are pregnant, you may not see any of the first 'product' to be made, but it is there. The first milk, colostrum, looks rather like melted butter. Sometimes it leaks out; sometimes not. There is no need to squeeze out or 'express' this colostrum unless you want to see what it is like.

More invisible activity

There are other preparations going on inside the breast as well. One of the first signs of pregnancy is sensitive breasts, and you may be aware of needing a different size bra. This is not just because the growing baby pushes out your rib cage. Inside your breasts, millions of tiny milk-making cells, complete with little muscles around groups of them ready to squeeze down the milk, as well as ducts ready to deliver the milk to your baby, are growing day by day. One writer described the inside of a woman's breast as looking like a well organised forest. Others picture it looking like cauliflower or bunches of tiny grapes.

It is the inside of the breast that makes and delivers the milk, and the nipple, with its 20 or so holes, like the rose of a watering can, which allows it out when the baby wants it. Later, at the touch of your baby's mouth, a hormone signals to the tiny muscles to push down more milk, while a second hormone instructs the breast's milk-making factory to speed up productivity in response to every 'delivery' of milk into the baby. The factory is now equipped with its own hormonal equivalent of information technology. It is responsive to your baby's needs, whether she is large, small, hungry, thirsty or even one of a pair.

Buying bras

Unless you have very neat breasts, and find the idea of wearing a bra even during breastfeeding very off-putting, you may want to prepare by buying bras for feeding, thinking about the ones you feel will suit you best, probably with opening fronts, wide straps, very adjustable fastenings, and with some way of keeping the whole thing in place while the baby feeds. It needs to be made of cotton for comfort, and preferably suitable for the end of pregnancy as well as afterwards. It may not be easy to get to the shops for a while once the baby is born. Again, talk to mothers who are breastfeeding and find out which bras they find the best. There are many different kinds available in shops. The NCT sells MAVA bras by mail-order service in a range of different styles – for a catalogue, write to NCT Maternity Sales (see page 197). In some areas there are agents who can fit you personally. These bras are suitable from five and a half months of pregnancy.

Plans and hopes

During pregnancy you will probably be thinking about how you hope your birth will be, perhaps by sharing ideas in classes, or reading about the choices you have in books. You may also be able to spend some time focusing on the first few breastfeeding experiences, so that you can begin thinking about how you want the feeding to go at the beginning, without having to do it when you are tired, or disorientated after the birth.

'I wish I had been stronger because I found out later that the nurse had settled him with a bottle of formula milk.'

Just as in birth plans it will help to be flexible, realising that not all births begin or end in a straightforward way. Similarly with breastfeeding, it is useful to know that however the first few hours after birth turn out, it is almost always still possible to breastfeed.

The areas you may like to think about, perhaps after you have read the chapter on starting breastfeeding, are your hopes for having the baby to hold right away, and to feed when the baby shows signs of being interested, and whether you want to breastfeed in the night. If you discuss this with whoever is going to be there supporting your birth, they will be able to remind you of your plans, and also act for you if, for example, you need a general anaesthetic. It is useful to get ready by finding out what the local policies are on breastfeeding. Most parents are now offered a visit around the unit in which their baby will be born and many hospitals also produce leaflets which outline their thinking on breastfeeding so that mothers can see how policy becomes practice. You may find, for instance, that only mid-wives, or those specially trained to do so, are able to offer breast-feeding advice, and that any extra fluid medically necessary will only be given (usually now by using a small cup rather than a bottle) after a discussion between yourself and a member of the medical staff. If extra fluid has to be offered, it is a good idea to watch someone who knows how to do this and then practise yourself in hospital if fluid is needed more than once. Basically the baby sits up on your knee, and the cup, at least half full, lies between her lips (just like when an adult drinks) so that she can feel the fluid and sip it. If fluid is poured into her mouth she may be worried and struggle. You may feel it would still be useful to have your wishes recorded to refer to in case your preferences are forgotten, for example during a busy shift change.

Afterwards you may like to write to the hospital with positive comments, as some parents do, together with any constructive suggestions. Sometimes a complaint may even be helpful in showing hospital management the need for more midwives.

Real motherhood

Everyone tries to tell you before you have a baby what a time-consuming job it is – that is why there are so many jokes about sleepless nights. It is unusual to get the chance to watch every moment of a normal day for a mother. Even when we visit a sister or a friend she may put off many jobs or have done them at 6am simply because we are coming. The fact that we are there changes things as well. We can rock a fretful baby while she cooks, or iron for her while she feeds the baby. We would need to be a 'fly on a wall' to see the reality of doing everything ourselves, and it may not be until you are mothering full time that you begin to understand the demands of the role.

Responsibility

Having a new person in the family asks a lot of those already in it. All new parents have a great many changes to cope with, and although breastfeeding is just one of them, it is one upon which much attention is focused. Not only is it important because it is a good way to keep the baby well and growing, but also it is one of the main tasks which a mother will be doing for several hours a day, with little training. From the birth, instead of asking 'How are you?' one of the new questions will be 'How is the feeding going?' Taking the sole responsibility for four months or so for continuing your baby's growth can feel quite a tall order. You have usually been able to do this for nine months already, however, and you do have others to help and support you. Fortunately, there are plenty of other ways, as well as checking on how much is going into the baby, of making sure all is well. Most of all as you prepare for the baby, it may help to be ready in your imagination for a small person who will need 24-hours-a-day care, however she is to be fed.

'I wasn't quite prepared for the round the clock nature of his demands.'

Imagining it all

As you become more aware of the baby inside you as a person, by feeling the tickles and kicks of her fingers and legs, and by seeing other people's reactions, you will begin to get a picture of 'after the birth'. It is very hard to imagine what breastfeeding a baby might be like, and much easier to imagine bottle-feeding, which most of us have done, either with real babies, or with dolls. When breastfed babies are shown on television it tends to be as famine victims in distant countries or in the context of debate about feeding outside the home, and we rarely see uneventful breastfeeding as part of normal family life. Perhaps it is even harder than imagining a real baby curled up small inside us ready to be born as a separate person.

Imagine yourself breastfeeding – what you see, or feel. Is it warm and cosy, or uncomfortable? Are other people there or not? Where are you sitting – by the television or fire in the living room, or in a bedroom? You may be lying down in bed, nice and relaxed. Many mothers find later that they are more able to breastfeed in public than they imagined. Try to think where the pictures may have come from and how true to life they might be for you. Your partner, parents, and in-laws may be willing to share the kind of pictures they have. Imagine how you would hold the baby – does she look like a baby who is just going to have a bottle popped into her mouth, on her back, or is she pulled up closely to your breast ready to take it into her mouth?

When you are thinking about feeding the baby, you might find it helpful to picture how things will be a few minutes after the baby is born, after an hour or so, then a week after the birth,

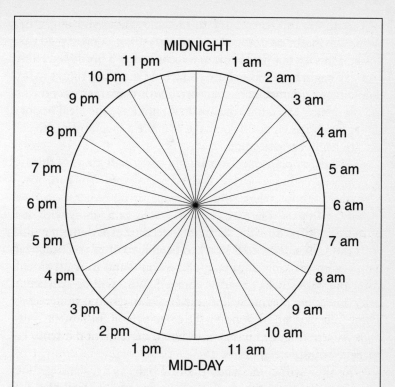

You could use a 24-hour clock like this to look at the way you spend your time before you have a baby – sleeping, eating, working, in leisure, talking time, and so on.

You might like to imagine how a new baby might affect your priorities – how do you imagine she might fit in or change things?

Friends with babies may be able to give you some ideas for probable timings of night feeds at the beginning of a baby's life, and the times you could expect a baby to wake up in the morning and so on. ALL BABIES ARE DIFFERENT THOUGH, SO YOU CANNOT KNOW WHEN YOURS WILL NEED YOU – and of course they do change in their needs from day to day.

Later, it may help to use the diagram if you are feeling you never have a moment to yourself, to get a realistic picture of how long your baby is spending crying, feeding, sleeping, and so on, and to look for any improvements.

and a month and so on. Try to imagine where you might be. What you might be doing about breastfeeding. As you read this book, if this is your first baby, or a second after a bottle-fed baby, you will begin to visualise how you would most like things to be. Sometimes circumstances, like needing a caesarean section or having a baby early, may mean you do not have the ideal opportunity you hoped for and you have to make a special effort to get help to begin breastfeeding.

It is hard to plan since you are not sure of all kinds of things. Not very many babies arrive on the day expected. You can, however, think about what your needs might be either as a new mother, with a baby to care for, as a couple, or a family with one or more children already. With breastfeeding especially in mind, you could consider who is likely to be able to offer you practical help – with cooking, shopping and so on – and to what extent you can lay in stocks of meals yourself. Who will be around to field 'intruders'? Who will remind you of things you know? These jobs may all be done by the same person for a while, perhaps your partner or mother or sister or a friend, or they may be parcelled out to neighbours.

The time will come when the real baby is here and getting hungry, so the next stage in the journey is to be equipped for the start.

CHAPTER TWO

Starting

'It eventually dawned on me that although I was by now cuddling my new arrival I'd completely forgotten about putting him to the breast.'

Being a newly delivered mother is an experience unlike anything else, and as the majority of women in this country will be away from home at this time, the sense of strangeness can be even greater. It can be quite overwhelming. It may be the first time, apart from a visit or two, that you have been in hospital and now you are a 'patient' – even though you are not ill. Many women wish to have a close person with them at this time, as well as the midwife who sees their baby into the world. The baby's father, if he is able to attend the birth, may also feel overwhelmed by the experience. After the baby has been delivered you are often alone for a while as a family: 'I'm very glad we didn't have anyone else around then because it was very special for us.' Once you have become acquainted with each other you may feel it is time for the first feed.

Many women will be helped with their first breastfeeding experience by someone who was there when the baby was born. If you are having a home delivery, your midwife can stay on for a while to help you begin breastfeeding, and she, or another community midwife, will then continue to return to help you further.

Different births

'Simon was born after a wonderful labour without drugs and after only being in hospital for an hour and a half. This time I felt much more in control of the situation . . . giving the baby a good feed before we left the delivery suite.'

Your birth sets the scene for the first breastfeed, even if this does not take place at the time. An unhurried birth with no complications may produce a tired but relieved mother ready to hold her baby while she waits for her to recover from the surprise of birth and show signs of hunger. Even if the birth is not straightforward, you may still feel exhilarated about your baby.

Many babies are not ready to feed straightaway, and are happy simply to lie in your arms, smelling and perhaps tasting you. This is an introduction for you both, giving you time to look at all the details of your baby, invisible inside you for so long. Her feet and hands are still blue and that is OK. Unless she is a bit late, or has been washed, she will still be smeary with protective white cream from inside the watery womb.

At some point soon after the birth you will currently be offered a first dose of vitamin K for you baby. The reasons for this should have been discussed with you before you had your baby. There is some evidence that vitamin K helps babies born with rare conditions or placed at risk by 'assisted' deliveriy to avoid damage from serious bleeding. Further doses will be offered during the first few months of life unless the first dose was given by injection. It may be possible to request that any oral vitamin K given at this time is not offered just before or just after the baby takes the breast, as the preparation tastes unpleasant and you may want your baby to remember being close to you as a time for getting something that tastes good. Your own milk does contain vitamin K, especially in the hindmilk and colostrum. At the time of writing, the Department of Health is preparing a leaflet about parents' choices around offering vitamin K to their babies.

'The birth involved gas and air, pethidine, a drip (my waters had broken and things were not progressing very quickly) and lastly an epidural, as I had been pushing for two hours and forceps were needed to turn him round. Afterwards I was on cloud nine.'

Observations made in Sweden of what a baby does if she is left against her mother's body after birth and disturbed as little as possible, shows that babies often follow a pattern of behaviour, at first lying quietly recovering from the birth and then beginning to lick their lips and move their hands to their mouths showing interest in reaching for the breast, which they find by smell.* Babies who are allowed to follow this built-in pattern often begin breastfeeding with very little difficulty, and the mother can feel she and the baby have made a good start together. There may be reasons for mother and baby to be separated briefly of course, and it is possible to recapture this opportunity later – skin to skin contact is especially helpful for this. However, many separations occur not out of medical necessity but out of habit – for example there is no need for the baby to be weighed before the first feed, and a mother can hold her baby even while having any stitches necessary. If the baby's father is present at the birth his special role can be to watch – and protect – this process, perhaps supporting you both together psychologically and even physically if you are shaky after the effort of birth. Most hospital policies now favour the first breastfeed being given while you are still in the delivery room, as this is a time when the baby may be alert and ready to feed. You can of course ask to wait for a while if you feel too shaky.

After such a period, even without feeding, babies often seem to recognise you again and will feed well when you next try. Even premature babies who have been tube-fed for weeks on end can learn to breastfeed, so do not panic if you are not able to get everything together immediately. 'All the breastfeeding literature that I had read told me that the baby would come out wanting to suck immediately. They don't all want to suck . . . to begin with he just wasn't hungry.'

If you have your baby by caesarean section with a spinal or epidural anaesthetic, then you will be able to hold and feed the baby but you may need to remain lying down for some hours afterwards. Furthermore, you may not have been able to eat for some time and so feel rather wobbly even lying down. If the operation is done under general anaesthetic, your partner or a midwife may be able to put the baby to your breast even while you are coming round, so she can begin to get to know you before you are introduced to her! Even if you have already fed one baby, this kind of scenario can shake your confidence, but the staff will be aware that you need extra help.

Your feelings about having had a non-vaginal delivery, or one needing varying degrees of medical intervention, do have some bearing on your approach to breastfeeding. All kinds of thoughts may come to you – that you must make up to the baby for a less than perfect start by being certain that the next stage is natural, or, however irrationally, that your body was not able to provide a normal delivery and so it may not be able to deliver or make milk properly either. You may just feel gratitude that the baby is here and that you can make a new start on an entirely different process. However you feel, it may help to talk over the birth itself with someone who will listen carefully to your feelings. You may also need to think about how the birth is physically affecting the way you are experiencing feeding. Perhaps you have painful stitches or a headache. Pethidine, often used to help with pain in labour, can leave your baby feeling sleepy and not fully able to get in touch with her instincts about how to breastfeed. It is worth discussing the (fairly long-lasting) effects of this drug with a midwife or antenatal teacher as you think about your birth plan. If you do find that both you and your baby are feeling too dozy to start breastfeeding while you are in the delivery room, with assistance you can still hold her so that she is used to your smell, and you can ask for help later with starting to breastfeed. Everyone may need to be patient through this process.

The birth: being a new baby

The baby too is going through a period of extreme change. Not only can she see new shapes and lights, and hear strange sounds, but after a while there is no food going into her tummy from you. She is usually born able to cope with a period of little food – think of the newborn babies in the Mexican earthquake who were the only ones to come out alive after days of being trapped – but at some time soon she will feel a new pain which overwhelms her and makes her cry: hunger.

Beginning to learn

Breastfeeding involves a new set of skills for a mother and baby to practise before they both feel comfortable and relaxed. The start of the experience could be compared with the first few lessons in a car. At first there seems to be so much to remember and to get right, and you can feel clumsy. Some people may take to the new experience like ducks to water, but many find it all rather bewildering. Mothers often remember their first breast-feed quite vividly, even if they are still fuzzy from a painkilling drug like pethidine.

It is more likely to feel as if labour was the driving test, and now you have to be responsible for the baby all by yourself. You will both be new to the experience and it is unlikely that there will be much time available for 'lessons', nor will they always be from the same person. Fortunately, you are not really alone in this journey – others are ready to help you both. To begin with, usually the mother, father or midwife will help the baby to the breast, possibly quite soon after the birth. Sometimes the baby is brought to you when you are in the ward. If you had an epidural or spinal anaesthetic, you will still have no pain after the birth, so this is a good time to try a first feed.

This book will look at the first feeds in slow motion. Every mother and baby makes an individual pair, but there are some basic principles that work well for almost all mothers and babies and which help you get off to a good start in breastfeeding.

Many of these principles are about getting the baby and you together. You will see and hear many words used for this impor-tant action – 'positioning' the baby at the breast, 'latching' her on, 'fixing' her, and so on. The tend to sound rather clinical and cold, but they all describe the way that your baby and your breast become really securely joined, until she or you actively choose to stop this hold. This is very different from bottle-feed-ing where the teat is 'plugged in'. One breastfeeding mother described her baby as being 'glued' to her breast, and it can look like this. This is so that the milk can transfer from you to her without any pain or unnecessary delay.

Because were are used to having to be in charge in new situ-ations and because we have all seen so much bottle-feeding, it is easy to imagine that somehow the task is to get the breast into the baby's mouth. One unhelpful habit in breastfeeding, which is connected to using bottles, is pointing the nipple at the baby and pushing it into her mouth. It may help to remember that the baby needs to *take* the breast. In fact, a 'primitive' woman probably delivered her baby by herself in a crouching position or on all fours and so moved the baby up to the breast from there herself. Some women now give birth in a similar position. Even if you are lying down, or sitting quite upright it is perhaps worth bearing in mind the upward movement of the baby in these circumstances, rather than remembering pictures that we may have of the baby being handed over by a nurse from above.

Take your time

The baby's suckling instinct is at its strongest during the hours and days after the birth, but it may not be her first reaction as she recovers from birth. One careful observer of babies, here and abroad, has noticed that alert babies who are not already crying for food may learn particularly well. Some will be eager to get on with this, others will not. Most babies are born still full of food from your placenta, and will not need more than the small amount of colostrum available during the first few days of life, so usually there is no rush to get any food into her immediately. The first feeds are to help you both to learn how to get together and to give some colostrum.

If you are still lying on the delivery table, the baby can be put beside or on top of you and you should be getting some help with positioning her at the breast. If you want help, ask for it if you are not offered it. Later, on the postnatal ward, or at home, sitting in a chair is a good place to continue learning as you may feel you have more control of the situation. But wherever you are, the basic principles still apply.

Starting with you

You need to be as comfortable as you can, whether lying down or sitting up. If you are sitting up in bed or on a chair, you need to be *quite upright*, propped with as many pillows or cushions as you need. Your baby will be on your lap, and this may feel too low for her to reach the breast without you lifting her up, so you

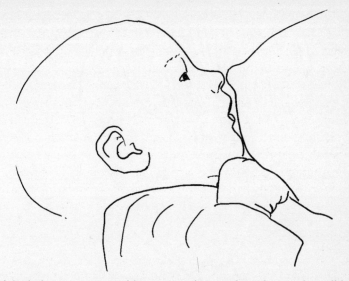

If the baby's nose is roughly opposite her mother's breast she will be able to respond to your touching her top lip with your nipple by opening her mouth and reaching up, taking in more of the breast from under the nipple than from above it.

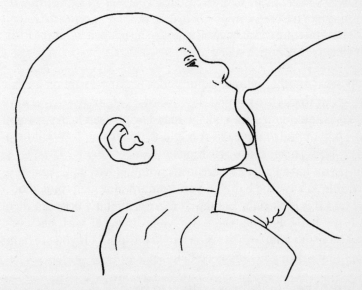

The baby's mouth is wide open and her tongue down so she can get a good mouthful of breast tissue where the milk lies waiting for her to stroke it out with her tongue.

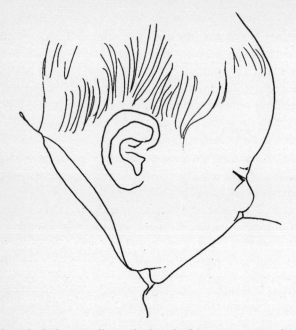

When the baby is well attached to the breast it may not be possible to see whether her lips are nicely folded back but you can see her chin is pushing into the breast. As you both become more experienced this will be something which happens quickly and without having to think about it.

may need another pillow to put under her. If you are on a chair and your thighs are sloping downwards, you may feel you have to keep hauling her up, and she may begin to get heavy for you and pull at your nipple, so something under you feet will help. Try a book, magazine or cushions.

If you have had a caesarean section you may find it uncomfortable to have the baby on your tummy, although some mothers find this is all right as long as there is a pillow between them and the baby. Feeding the baby lying down, or with her body tucked under your arm are alternative positions . If you are hampered by a drip you may need help.

Where to have the baby in relation to you
Make sure that the baby is turned to face you, with her tummy against yours. If she is on her back, like a baby expecting a

bottle, she will have to turn her head to reach you. This is uncomfortable both for her (try drinking over your shoulder to see why) and for you: she may end up having to tug on your nipple to keep it in her mouth.

Babies feel rather floppy at first, and immediately after birth are also rather wet and slithery, so you need to hold them close to you all the way along their bodies. They also wave their arms around when they are worried – another good reason to feed while they are alert but not desperately hungry. One of the baby's arms can be tucked down out of the way under your breast. This is easier when she is on her side.

Whatever position you adopt, aim to have the baby's nose roughly opposite your nipple so that she can let her head fall back a little as she reaches it up to scoop in a good mouthful of breast tissue from below the nipple – which lies in the top half of her mouth above her tongue. You may understand better how this position works if you try to get hold of the fleshy part of the base of your thumb as you hold your hand facing you with that part opposite your mouth. You will find you can only get a bit of yourself into your mouth whereas if you try lifting it up above your mouth, you have to come 'up and under'. This way you get a much bigger mouthful of your own thumb base. Similarly, the baby gets a much more useful mouthful of breast tissue if she makes this kind of movement. Where the baby's face is exactly will depend on the shape and size of your breasts and how they are placed on your body – high or low – and on how your nipples are set, centrally on the breast or slightly out to the side, and so on. If you are sitting up, the baby's head usually need not be as far out as the crook of your arm – this is where she would need to be to accept a bottle.

Your breast

If you support your breast by holding your hand against your ribs beneath it, you will see that you can make a nice plump shape for the baby to attach herself to. If, usually later, you feel your breast is very heavy and 'floppy', you may want to cup your hand underneath it, but make sure that your thumb is well away from the nipple and the areola around it. Your whole hand needs to be far back, so that you cannot try to make a kind of bottle and teat out of your breast to poke into the baby's mouth. This would reduce the amount of breast tissue she can get hold of, limiting her intake of milk.

'Scissoring' the breast – holding it with two fingers – is common but not helpful unless you absolutely need to do it, if for example you cannot see the baby because you are blind.

Your arms

Whether she is lying beside you or on your lap, you need to support her bottom and top half, so that her ear, shoulder and hip are in a straight line. Some mothers feel most comfortable holding their babies so that they lie against their arm on the same side as the breast they are going to feed from, and they can then reach across with the opposite hand to support the breast if it needs it. Others prefer to use the hand on the same side as the breast to support it, and to support the baby's back against their other forearm. Once the baby is on the breast, you may then like to use the arm on the same side as the breast you are feeding from to cradle her.

Your hands

There is no need to hold the back of her head – your fingers can just come up the side of her neck behind her ears. Babies do not like having their heads held, and this also tends to push her face *down* towards your breast, whereas you are aiming to make sure that, when she arrives on your breast, she is slightly reaching back with her head *up* to your breast. At first it does feel as if you need at least three arms, one to support the baby, one to support the breast and one to move the baby's arms out of the way, or help to move the baby to the breast. It seems unbelievable that eventually you will have a hand free to answer the phone.

Interesting the baby in the breast

The baby has a 'rooting' reflex which helps her to turn to find the breast and then open her mouth to suckle. Some babies open their mouths really well quite quickly; others take time to do it.

Very gently tickle her top lip with your nipple to encourage her to open her mouth wide. The harder you push, the more she is likely to make a quick and inaccurate grab for your breast, so take your time and let her learn to open really wide. There is no rush. She needs to take the nipple, and lots of breast tissue into her mouth, reaching back to milk the milk sacs. These are the widened places inside your breast near the ends of the milk ducts, just beneath the edge of your areola.

When you feel that she is really gaping her mouth as wide open as a big yawn, move her towards you so that her mouth comes up to the breast. It will be the whole baby you move in a straight line, not just her head. Her chin needs to reach the breast first and stay in close contact with it, as it is her lower jaw which supports her tongue as it does the work of milking the breast tissue.

Safe inside the baby's mouth

Your nipple makes about one third of what is inside the baby's mouth. This means it is safe inside her and not scraping in and out, or being squeezed by her gums. It reaches back to the baby's soft palate. If you feel your own soft palate, behind the hard top of your mouth – much bigger of course than your baby's – you can see how soft and safe a place this is, so let as much as possible be enclosed. It may help to be leaning forwards slightly so that your breast drops towards the baby as she comes up. Her tongue does not rasp up and down your nipple either, but a wave of muscle movement presses from the tip of her tongue to its back, smoothing out the milk she has squeezed down from the milk sacs.

It may be that the first open mouth is not quite wide enough. Or you may miss the first opportunity. There is no need to panic. Your baby has shown you she can do it or that she can do it better! You can let the baby fall gently back a few inches after touching her lips again to remind her what to do. Dabbing her mouth quickly with the nipple may not give her the time she needs to remember what to do. You can see why it may help to work on this while your baby is not already crying for food; this way she is less likely to get upset. Watch out for her rooting or moving her lips and turning towards you and try then. Having her skin to skin can also help the whole thing to work better. You can practise while she is sleeping. What nicer than to come round in your mother's arms and find food, drink and comfort waiting for you?

When her mouth is very wide open, it fits against your breast. In some women, the whole areola disappears inside the baby's mouth. This depends on the size of your areola – if it is quite big, then you still see some of it, especially at the top. If it is small, even the whole lot disappearing might not be quite enough to give the baby a really good mouthful.

The baby's tongue fills up part of the bottom of her mouth ready to make a little trough around the nipple and breast tissue and her mouth needs to be aimed so that she gets more areola from below the nipple into her mouth than from above. The baby reaches up like someone eating an apple dangling above them on a string, taking more of the areola below the nipple than above it – the nipple is not central in her mouth.

You can leave the baby on the first breast you offer for as long as she likes, as long as she is not hurting you. This may be only a few minutes or a long feed of say half an hour. Then she may want to have some colostrum or milk from the other side. Pauses during feeding are normal in breastfeeding. The first feeling of your baby on the breast can be quite powerful. Her jaws are made to milk efficiently and strongly, but after a few moments this should not feel painful.

Checking it is all right

Someone else can look at the baby and make sure that her bottom lip is curled downwards, showing how wide open her mouth is. (If you do this yourself, it is possible you may disturb her good position.) The baby's tongue *under* the nipple may be seen as she comes off the breast. Her chin is somewhat less prominent than yours, to fit snugly up to the breast and allow the jaws and tongue to work there, and should be close in too.

'The midwife helped us to get latched on, and the power of that first suck nearly took my breath away.'

There is no need to pull back your breast from her nose. Babies have specially shaped nostrils which look very different from yours and allow them to have their faces quite close to the breast without any problems. Babies who cannot breathe have the sense to stop feeding and come off the breast. If you feel she may be having difficulties, try pulling her bottom half in towards you. If you imagine the baby like a see-saw with uneven ends, and your breast in her mouth as the pivot, you will see that when you pull in her bottom half, the top of her head will automatically swing out.

If it is wrong

Whether it is you or a health professional helping the baby to the breast, if it is done with the aim of pushing the areola skin and the nipple *into* the baby, rather than persuading the baby to use her own good reflexes to take the breast, it may well not work: 'It seemed that every nurse on the ward helped jam his mouth around my nipple but he would soon come off . . . one week later we were released from hospital with a bag of creams for *very* sore nipples and a hungry baby.'

'I couldn't get him to latch on at all – every time he opened his mouth and I popped my breast in, he clamped shut and out it slid.'

If there is continual pain as you feed, rather than just for the initial surprising moments, or if you know the position is wrong in another way, use your little finger to break the strong suction which the baby uses to hold your breast in her mouth. If it goes on hurting, and your nipples continue to feel sore between feeds, this is most likely to be a sign that the position needs to be better, and you should get skilled help. It may also help to look back at the section 'Beginning to learn' starting on page 25. There is no one magically right position for all babies and women; another tiny bit further on may make all the difference to a miserable baby or mother. Your fingers, or anyone else's, in the way, trying to 'point the end', will make things worse. The wide open mouth with the baby's tongue down over her bottom gums is the main aim. If your baby seems to want to push her tongue up rather than letting it fall down over her bottom lip it may help to show her slowly what to do. It has been found that babies held in front of an adult will, at a young age, imitate what they see – putting out their tongues for instance, so this may well be worth trying. If you can, try to get someone to watch a feed right from this stage to when the baby falls asleep or spits you out to show a really satisfying feed. Just a quick look may not give enough information as it is not always easy to see when the breast is generously full of milk and the baby has her chin nicely pushing into a soft breast.

The way it works

Other information about breastfeeding may be useful in getting it to work for you. Some aspects raised here are researched and some are practical knowledge which women have found out for themselves.

Beginning with the baby

The baby's stomach is very small at birth – about the length of your thumb – and is ready to receive colostrum in small quantities – she is not designed to take large feeds right away or always have both breasts. Her stomach slowly stretches like a balloon to take milk in larger amounts.

Colostrum is available in small quantities – as precious as caviare. It is the special milk which is first on offer to the baby and is a combination of food and protective proteins which line the baby's digestive system, while she builds up her own immunity. It also helps to prevent jaundice by speeding up the passage of the baby's first motions, called meconium.

From around the third or fourth day after the baby is born, colostrum is gradually diluted by breastmilk. The afterbirth leaving your body triggers this change. A whole range of milks is then available, in varying proportions according to the baby's needs, but always in the same order in each breast. This is like a gradual progression from skimmed milk, by way of semi-skimmed, to silver top. Unlike formula milk, no feeds are homogenised, with the cream spread evenly. This is an à la carte menu for the baby, who chooses for herself the quality as well as the quantity of mil, to have at each feed. It is rather like offering a glass of juice before a meal, and moving on through thin soup to the even more filling part of a nourishing dinner. Fortunately, experience, confirmed by research, has shown that your baby can manage all the details of ordering and eating each meal, depending on her needs for fluid and food, and so there is no need to worry about interfering in any way with how much is eaten or drunk. All you need to do is let the baby go on feeding from the first side you offer, until she chooses to come off, and either take the other side or call it a day. It is a good idea always to offer the other breast in case the baby does want another whole balanced menu or just a 'cup of tea' to wash down what she had on the first side. Making sure that the baby has finished at the first breast at a particular feed does not mean that the first side is 'finished' or empty. In fact, it is impossible to empty the breast as the next order begins to be made while feeding is still going on.

Even if we do interfere by timing the feeds, in the old-fashioned way, so that the baby gets two 'juices' first (by offering two short feeds, one on each breast) the baby will actually start to reorganise things after a while to get at the creamier milk. It seems a pity to try to confuse the system, when the baby can do it all without clocks.

Let-down

You are well designed too. As the breast grows heavier in pregnancy, a nice rounded surface under the nipple is ready for the baby to grasp and milk. Not only do you make and offer milk, you also possess the ability to allow your milk to flow to the baby: this is the let-down reflex. It causes tiny muscles in your breast to squeeze down milk every time your baby feeds (and sometimes in between). You can see the baby on the front cover of this book helping the mother to let her milk down by dimpling her breast with a warm hand. Let-down generally happens a minute or so after the beginning of the feed, though it is quite normal for it to take longer, giving the baby a chance to take the foremilk which is lying ready in the breast. It is quite hard to stop it from happening. Even when your baby is not feeding, and you just hear her or someone else's baby crying, or think about feeding her, you may see milk leaking out, or feel it surging warm or tingling inside your breasts. Some women never feel this sensation or only grow to be aware of it later in feeding:

' "The let-down reflex is quite strong isn't it?" – what feeling was my friend describing? I felt nothing – ever.' Others find it very strong.

'In the early weeks especially, I often found let-down really painful. I can remember saying through clenched teeth that the books said some women could reach orgasm while breastfeeding, but it didn't feel much like that to me.'

You can see it happening not only if you leak – again not a universal experience – but best of all when you notice the baby's suckling change from the fast, eager nibbling sucks at the beginning of a feed to the deep, once-a-second gulps or sighs of really good swallowing.

It is known that the process of let-down can be affected by extreme anxiety, for example, so that for a few moments if you are very worried or frightened, the milk may not flow quite so quickly from the breast to the baby. Once she has got the first milk which was waiting in the sacs and ducts there may be a pause while she works hard to stimulate your let-down. This does not mean that if you get worried or upset the milk will magically disappear. It just means that the powerful hormone adrenalin is stopping the let-down reflex from working at the moment, in case there was something you needed to run away from, or fight with, without letting milk out of your breasts. Most of our worries and fears nowadays are not ones we need to run from or fight about, but it may help to talk to someone to relieve the loneliness of your worry, or have a good cry, or do some relaxation – sighing away the tension – until the milk is able to flow.

Milk flow

The famous doctor Truby King, a fairly typical 'expert' in the earlier years of this century, decided that women should not allow anyone to speak to them while they were feeding, as this might affect the flow of milk. Many women who feed their babies during happy conversations with friends, partners and children would resent such solitary confinement.

Fears about not having enough milk are still common today, reflected in the numbers of women who gave this as their reason for stopping breastfeeding in the first few weeks. The research which explains so clearly about the baby's demand ordering the mother's supply seems really difficult to get over. Perhaps it is partly because anyone who has not fed a baby finds it hard to imagine actually making milk – even while you are doing it you may feel this yourself. If you should find you don't have enough milk it is very unlikely to be because you are unlucky enough to have defective breasts.

One of the ways to make sure mothers do not have enough milk is to stop them from offering the breast to their babies freely, for long enough or often enough. You probably know that ten minutes a side and four-hourly feeding began to be routine in the 1940s and 1950s and so you can see how easily people get the idea that there was something wrong with a lot of women, since it almost inevitably led to a shortfall, and probably it was women who 'cheated' who were the ones to keep going. Babies born at the turn of the century are considerably less likely to suffer from such unhelpful rules.

As milk is being taken, and the baby's mouth is simulating the breast, a hormone sends a message – 'Make more for the next feed.' This is not at all like bottles of milk where, if we drink it all freely, we end up without any, but much more like the filling up of a lavatory cistern in response to use. Using bottles or extra fluid of any kind sends a message to make less next time. A protein in breastmilk left in the breast stops too much being manufactured. Another way of visualising the way that breastfeeds follow one another is to think of those silk handkerchiefs that magicians pull out of their pockets. They knot the corner of each carefully around the last one so that the procession of multi-coloured silk flows out. Similarly, as you feed you are making it possible for the next meal to be ready for your baby in an unbroken chain until you or the baby decide to end the flow.

Another way that mothers can end up with babies who are not getting enough milk is where babies are not well attached to the breast and so do not manage to take enough of what is on offer either to grow well, or to place an order for the next meal.

The baby and mother together

You can see that breastfeeding works best where there are responses on both sides. Just as breast and baby need to fit together physically, so the mother needs to respond to the baby's needs – for a drink, or a long feed, or two short feeds close together, or a time for comforting herself – whatever the baby is wanting.

The baby helps *you* too, as suckling reduces blood loss after birth, helps ease out nipples which are not perfectly ready and prevents your breast from getting engorged (uncomfortably full of milk and other fluids). If you were able to feed on the delivery table this may have helped push out the afterbirth. She will still need feeding in the night: it is then that the milk-making hormone prolactin is at its highest level. This helps you to establish a good supply so that later she can begin to work towards night sleeps.

On the postnatal ward

For most mothers, being back on the postnatal ward can feel very uncomfortable after the hard delivery bed, and labour of birth. You now have a time to practise the new skills of breast-feeding together. One second-time mother sent us extracts of a journal of her breastfeeding experiences: 'Alice was born eight hours ago by caesarean section, and we've not seen each other since then. Now she's hungry and I'm nervous – will she know instinctively what to do? Can I remember?

. . . Well, I've done it! An understanding midwife busied herself in the vicinity just in case we needed help, but Alice latched on as though she'd done it all before. It seemed so natural to tuck this little bundle under my arm and yet I always fed Jenny across my lap.'

Special beginnings

Twins

If you have had twin babies you will have extra work right from the beginning. It can be harder to fall in love with two at once, and, sadly, it is more likely that they will be born slightly early and so have to spend some time in a Special Care Baby Unit. It

Reminders of what you can both do

You and the baby both bring to this new experience of breast-feeding a mixture of useful instincts and learnable skills

The baby can:

- feel hungry and cry to tell you
- 'root' for the breast
- learn to smell your breastmilk and turn to you
- open her mouth very wide
- breathe through her nose – even close to your breast
- milk the breast, swallow and breathe
- decide when she has had enough of one side
- decide if she needs the other side too
- decide when to stop feeding
- decide when she wants more

You can:

- respond to signs that she is ready to feed, such as turning her head for food – the last sign is crying, but you do not have to wait for that
- respond to her cries
- take her into your arms
- respond to the touch of the baby's mouth with your nipple
- learn to offer her your breast to that she can take a good mouthful
- let down your milk when you feel the warmth of her mouth
- keep making milk to meet her needs

can be useful to know something about expressing milk, just in case this is necessary for a little while (see Chapter 12).

Premature and ill babies

If, for any reason, your baby is in a Special Care Baby Unit you need to ask about expressing milk as soon as you can if you want your baby to have it and to go on to breastfeed. It may feel very sad and strange to be a mother without her baby when all the others have theirs, but you should be able to visit your special baby as soon as you are able to get out of bed. Chapter 12 looks at expressing, and there is more about complicated starts to breastfeeding in Chapter 4.

Why do we need to know all this?

Women who breastfeed successfully in other, less urbanised, countries do not know the names of milk-making hormones, or the exact fat content of milk. They can turn to many more mothers and grandmothers, with vast stores of personal experiences, if breastfeeding seems temporarily to suffer some kind of setback. Here, however, we have had nearly a hundred years of bottle-feeding, which confuses the issue greatly. For instance, formula is the same all the way down the bottle, and this easily becomes what we expect of all milks for babies. It is easy to think as well that as there is only one bottle used each feed, while there are two breasts ready, half a feed should come out of one and half out of the other, or that we might use one at once, rather than following the baby's requests which will vary from feed to feed, and day to day. Rules tend to come from thinking about bottle-feeding, and these are almost always unhelpful.

Mothers who hear explanations about the way breastfeeding really works, will often say 'I wish I had known that' or 'that explains it!' They may have wondered why a baby being offered two short feeds of foremilk was hard to settle and wanted very frequent feeds. It is not that there was anything wrong with the mother, or the baby, but that rules imposed from the outside made her uneasy about what she was doing. She was following the custom of automatically dividing a feed into two halves. So the baby got two 'drinks', felt too full, and was quickly hungry.

Before learning to drive, you already have useful abilities, like guessing what moving objects are likely to do next and being able to use your arms to steer something less worrying than a car. You just need to apply them to the new situation. As with driving, starting (and stopping, which we come to later) is one of the hardest parts. A lot is happening to you and to the baby. You have the instincts and skill-learning potential which you need for breastfeeding: for both experiences, you need encouragement, self-confidence and good teaching.

CHAPTER THREE

Straightforward starts

'I held him to my breast desperately, aware that I hadn't a clue what I was doing but equally desperate to hold him and feel his body and know he was all mine.'

When you have had your baby and are back in the postnatal ward, you may find that although you are tired, it is very hard to sleep. This is common after birth and this is a good time to get used to your baby. She too may be awake and even if she is not demanding food, this can be a good time to begin practising breastfeeding in a calmer setting: 'Sheila was born at home and went to the breast immediately. She suckled well. In hospital with her brother I was not allowed to bring him into bed with me and lost lots of sleep feeding. With Sheila at home we spent most of the nights together in the early days.'

You may go home quite quickly and have very little to do with the life of a hospital ward, but many mothers spend some days there with their first baby. You will meet a lot of different helpers, each with their own ideas about how best to help you. Most hospitals are working hard to get a consistent policy on breastfeeding, and to find ways in which health professionals can let each know what previous helpers have suggested.

Mealtimes in hospital are often much earlier than we are used to at home, and as well as caring for the baby, there is a lot of other activity, like your physiotherapy and having visitors. You may find it hard to sleep in a strange bed, with babies making even quiet noises as they sleep.

Your first breastfeeds may feel fairly public, unless you are in a single room, perhaps after a caesarean. Being in a ward does mean that you are more likely to be able to catch someone's eye for some help, but you can, of course, also summon it. This will be especially necessary if you cannot yet get out of bed, or lift the baby yourself.

'The situation was not helped by the fact that I was very self-conscious about being seen breastfeeding by male members of my family.'

Some women prefer to try out the first steps of feeding with the curtains around the bed, so that they are able to concentrate without others distracting them or watching them working on positioning the baby: 'in a busy ward with visitors coming in and out, a nervous awkward first-time mum becomes terrified and loses complete confidence.' For others, it lightens the tension to be aware of other mothers, or even talk through what is happening with an experienced breastfeeder. You can ask for curtains to be drawn around you or pulled back, whichever you feel most comfortable with at the time. Sometimes it is nice to start in private and, when the baby and you have got the hang of it more, to rejoin the rest of the ward.

If you or the baby get frustrated as you work at feeding, stop trying for a while, and calm the baby, and yourself. Talk to the baby about what is happening. You may like to try another position or do something quite different altogether.

Why it all can seem rather confusing

The advice given to you when learning to breastfeed can feel like having three or four different people trying to see you out of a tight corner in a car park. They are all waving their arms in different ways while you try to decide who to trust. One reason is that the situation is changing, so what was suggested for the days when the baby was sleepy and you had colostrum, may seem very different from ideas for the day when your milk arrives, and the baby may be hungry all the time. Of course, it can be helpful to be offered alternatives to see which approach helps you.

Some midwives may give you a choice of things to try, which they know sometimes help mothers. But you may not feel free to choose what suits you best as each person helping can give the impression that their way is the only way.

'Although the staff were wonderful and I could never praise them highly enough, they all had slightly different ways, so at each shift change I was doing something different.'

Mothers may find that staff have different ideas for helping problems like sore nipples, for example. For this reason, it can be good to know the basics for yourself (see pages 25–34), so that you can work out what seems to be the most helpful advice. If a midwife is using the Royal College of Midwives book, *Successful Breastfeeding*, she may be able to show you how the research backs up her practice or point out the relevant part of the hospital's own policy on infant feeding to explain what is being done.

In many hospitals now, policies and practices have improved in line with research so that, for example, complementary feeds and bottle-feeds in the night are not automatically given to babies without a great deal of discussion between medical staff and the mother. It is now understood that nothing but breast-milk is normally needed. You may wish to weigh any benefits of giving formula against concerns about setting off a sensitivity to cow's milk in your baby, especially if there are allergies in your family on either side.

Even sucking water from a bottle may interfere with the learning about suckling which you and the baby are working hard on. Extra feeds of water have been found actually to reduce the amount of fluid taken overall by the baby.* If you are told that it is really necessary to give something extra, offering fluid by a cup or spoon is quite possible.

Another welcome disappearance is the insistence on regular and limited feeding times. The idea about feeding for ten minutes came from the average length of time a baby took to finish half a bottle-feed. If a baby is made to wait, crying, for a set time, she may be too distressed to feed properly – it is difficult sometimes to convince a screaming baby that the breast is there for her. If she is woken at someone else's 'right' time she may not be ready to feed. Only in Special Care Baby Units will babies be roused to feed at regular intervals. If a baby gets the message that the time available for feeding is always limited she may begin to feed in a hurried way and grab your breast fast. Limiting the times at the breast does not help sore nipples. As long as the position is right, the baby can feed for as long as she needs. If it is not, even a short feed will make the nipples sore.

In general, rules are disappearing – mothers can choose when to change nappies, and are not forced to swaddle their babies to feed and so on. At one time, all mothers had to fill in a chart, simply modified from the bottle-fed babies' charts, recording minutes instead of ounces. There are many problems with this as it is difficult to know whether to count the normal pauses as sucking or not, and all babies take milk – and all mothers deliver it – at different rates. Ten minutes might be plenty for one baby, and totally inadequate for another. With a more relaxed atmosphere, it is possible to give staff more accurate feedback about how long and how often little babies really do feed, when allowed to do so, and in this way to help the helpers to get a truer picture.

'I vowed I would not get hung up on rights and wrongs, routines, bottles of water, juice, and other spurious liquids.'

What to expect –
What is OK and what isn't

All babies are individuals with unique finger-prints. They have different patterns of suckling, swallowing and resting during feeds, and so will approach breastfeeding in all kinds of ways. Babies often pause after a burst of enthusiastic suckling to wait for milk to be let-down, and just to take a breather, like us during a meal. Because mothers and babies vary so much, it can be unhelpful to compare yourself with the woman in the bed opposite, but there are reassuring signs to look for.

Your baby may well sleep very well after a good feed of colostrum which gives you the chance to rest too, but some babies want to feed frequently from the word go. They may want up to 12 or more times on the breast during each 24-hour period. Some of these will be 'proper' feeds, and some will feel like shorter between-meals 'drinks' when the milk arrives.

The baby may be eager in feeding, at least for the first part of the feed, with strong jaw movements, and visible movements around her temples as she feeds. She will be alert, not listless, waiting until she has had some minutes of good feeding before usually falling asleep, looking drunk. A good feed on one side could easily last around half an hour. She may sometimes push the breast away with her tongue after a good feed. After a while you may notice little blisters on her lips – these are normal, do not hurt her and will go away on their own.

What goes in must come out

A baby passes little urine for the first 12 to 24 hours. After that, you might expect a couple of wet nappies for two or three days until your milk comes in Modern nappies are very absorbent and it may be difficult to tell how wet each one is. You can take one to bits to see what the filling is like dry and what it is like wet to give you a clue as to what is happening. You may then find your baby needing up to six to eight terry nappies, or five or six disposables each day. The baby's urine should be clear, colourless or very pale yellow, and not smelling of anything much at all.

The baby's first dirty nappies are quite a surprise with black sticky stuff called meconium, which the colostrum helps to clear out quickly. As letting it lie in the baby's insides can lead to an increased chance of jaundice this is a really good reason to give lots of colostrum feeds if the baby is cooperative. When your milk arrives, this meconium will change over a day or so to the usual breastfed baby's motion, which is also quite a new experience for most parents. It is rather like the consistency of scrambled egg and can be more liquid – indeed, it is surprisingly watery, especially if you see it happening. It varies from the colour of mustard (English, German or French) to a sunflower yellow, perhaps with little white curds, or occasional green streaks.

Meconium may take a little longer to clear after a caesarean delivery. Hospital staff will be keeping an eye on what comes out too, and you can ask about anything you are worried about.

Babies may take in air as well as milk around the time they are feeding – for example if they have to cry loudly – although a baby who is thoroughly 'glued' to her mother is much less likely to get wind in this way. As babies lie down a lot, wind tends to go downwards rather than come up and seems to cause some babies a bit of distress. Sitting them upright, or over your shoulder and rubbing gently or just waiting is usually enough. If nothing happens, don't worry, and there is no need to pat vigorously. Sometimes, a bit of milk comes up on top of the bubble of air so a cloth in the right place can be a good idea.

Once the milk has arrived

Anything like eight or twelve feeds a day is to be expected after the arrival of milk, so they might be two hours apart on average, perhaps with a little bit longer at night. It can be hard to count though, with little short drinks running into each other. Times between feeds vary enormously from perhaps one hour to as long as eight, although such long gaps may only happen once near the beginning.

Growing

Some weight loss is usual in hospital, as babies use up the special fat deposits laid down while they were in the womb. Up to ten per cent of the baby's birth weight is expected to be lost. Some babies, however, especially if they are demand fed, do not lose weight. Rather than thinking of a set date by which birthweight must have been regained, the upturn is usually looked for some time soon after your milk comes in.

It is impossible to know what kind of weight gain your baby wants to have. If both her mother and father are slightly built it is unlikely that she will be trying to be large, for instance.

More about positioning

It is a good idea to get the position of your baby right now while you have time to think, and help at hand. This will be the basis for the months of feeding ahead. It may help to look back over the positioning section on pages 25–34.

From above, it can be hard to tell how well the baby is taking the breast. Someone else, looking at the drawing on pages 27–28, may be able to see if the baby is taking a big enough mouthful of your breast with a wide enough mouth, especially if they are able to watch the 'approach'. Looking for curled back lips may not be easy, and no one should try to 'look' with their fingers in case they disturb things which are going well. Fortunately there are other ways to know if the baby is well positioned – these are outlined in the box overleaf. If the baby is really well attached you may be able to move your supporting hand away, though if your breasts are heavy or engorged this may still prove quite a challenge to the baby.

It is very easy to concentrate just on what we can see – the surface of the breast, especially the nipple and areola – perhaps because these are the parts which have changed most to the naked eye during pregnancy. It may help to think how a cushion cover can easily fail to fit well around the stuffing at one corner. What the baby needs to be able to do is get a really good mouthful of the tissue of the breast – the cushion's stuffing – inside and behind the nipple and areola, which is why it is no good just taking the skin and cramming it into the baby's mouth.

We can see how much is going into the baby from a bottle, but we need more faith to know it is going in from a breast. You can listen to it being gulped down and sometimes see it oozing out around the baby's mouth or dripping from you, but your body is careful with its resources and later you may notice little milk escaping. What you are most likely to see, because it flows most freely, is the foremilk, the useful thirst-quencher which looks thin and sometimes blueish. To see the white and creamy hindmilk, you may need gently to express a drop of milk at the end of a feed.

Position checklist

Is the baby:

- turned to you on her side?
- is her nose opposite your nipple?
- opening her mouth really well?

Are you:

- offering her a nice rounded breast without fingers shaping the end?
- moving all of her towards you so that she gets a good mouthful of breast tissue?
- holding her so she can let her head move up to the breast?

Can you see:

- the muscles at the side of her face by her ears moving as she suckles (not her cheeks being pulled in as if she was sucking on a teat)?
- her jaw moving against your breast working at breastfeeding?

Can you hear:

- the fast sucks change after a minute or more to deeper glugs?

Can you feel:

- no pain right through the feed?

The two signs that matter most if you are trying to tell whether things are going well are that you feel comfortable (even if you have had pain earlier, it should be improving) and that the baby is relaxed and swallowing milk.

Your feelings

How you feel about feeding may depend on what you are usually like. If you are a pessimist, even though you had a good birth, you may feel that breastfeeding will be bound to go wrong to make up for that. If you were disappointed in the way you gave birth, you may begin by expecting breastfeeding to be hard too. If you have always said to yourself that 'everything will be all right', then a less than perfect birth may have shaken your confidence badly, and a good birth may leave you unprepared for any slight problem. You may be confident and have your optimism questioned by others. Fortunately, the baby is just hungry and does not seem to know any gloomy thoughts you or others have.

You may find yourself crying for little real reason and be reassured by staff that this is quite usual, the 'third day blues' which are possibly hormonally caused. Do not worry that being upset will curdle the milk, stop your let-down or frighten the milk supply away. Millions of women down the years must have wept over their baby's heads as they came to realise how perfect, or how fragile or how not quite right they are, and have not starved them because of it. If you are tense, it is useful to talk to your baby, as well as others, and let out some of your distress or joy. Mothers can find that as tears flow, so does the milk.

Engorgement

When your milk comes in, any time between the second and fifth day after your baby is born, your breasts may feel very full, hot and tense. They are not only filling with milk but reacting to hormonal changes by an increasing blood and lymph supply, making them swollen. The more you are able to feed the baby in the good position you are working on, the more she will relieve enough of the tension for you to find this stage not too uncomfortable. It will go away by itself in about 24 hours. If this is a problem, see page 53 for ways to help. When your milk is beginning to come it may be useful to think about learning a simple way of expressing milk by hand (if you have not already done so) – not just because expressing can help you to relieve some pressure but also because it can be useful later. There is a description of an easy way to do this on page 159. Leaflets are available on expressing milk from the NCT, and many hospitals now have Baby Friendly information about expressing.

Comfort

Check that your shoulders are not aching because you are leaning over the baby in an uncomfortable position. Imagine someone touching them gently as you feed to remind you to let go of any tension. If you are uncomfortable while feeding, ask for help. Midwives have lots of ideas for sore areas, not just painkillers, but ice packs for bad bruising and painful stitches after the birth for example.

As you feed the baby, you may notice there is an increase in the amount of blood lost, and perhaps sensations of tightening in the area of your womb, known as afterpains. They are less usual with first than subsequent children, and vary in how strongly they are felt. If they are bad, you can ask for painkillers. Some women do not feel them at all and the good news is that after a few days the pain will go, and either you will be left with no sensations or pleasurable ones which are quite normal, though rarely discussed, and come as a bonus for the breastfeeding mother.

If you find breastfeeding painful for just a few moments at the beginning of a feed, this should pass. If it lasts all the way through a feed or you can see that the damage seems not to be healing then seek some professional help.

At the end of your first week with your baby, you may like to look back to see how your ideas of life at one minute, one hour and one week fit with reality. It can be useful to realise where you were right with your guesses, how much your expectations and reality differ, and how far being a parent is new territory.

CHAPTER FOUR

More complicated beginnings

'I felt completely geared up for the pain of labour and as a result felt I could handle it, but no one had said "breastfeeding can be really painful at first, but stick with it because it will become much easier".'

Sadly, there are many small ways in which your first few days of feeding can fail to get off to the perfect start which you may have hoped for or imagined. Sometimes your needs and the baby's do not quite 'fit' for a day or so. You may find that you are wide awake while the baby may want to sleep off the birth; you may be feeling sore and longing to rest and the baby may be very hungry, or you may feel very full of milk while the baby is sound asleep.

These mismatches can be upsetting so ask for help. What can seem like minor problems compared with a mother who has a baby in Special Care, for example having a sleepy jaundiced baby when you are engorged, can combine to make breastfeeding quite difficult. Try to be patient with the baby, and with yourself, and see the first few days as a learning period.

You may also find that you feel you cannot do as you would at home: 'I wanted to look at him and get to know him. However, in my dazed state and also being terrified of upsetting the staff, I didn't really dare argue.' In the next chapter about getting and using help, there are some ideas for asking for what you want without having to have a big argument.

What they all warn
you about – sore nipples

'Most of the books I read on the subject seem to dismiss sore nipples as a fairly minor problem which could be quickly and easily overcome. This was not what I experienced. During the first few days, even weeks, it made my relationship with the baby more difficult. I am sure that if I had been less determined I would have given up breastfeeding at a very early stage because of the agony it involved. As it was I breastfed Rachel for 15 months.'

Sore nipples do hurt. The wind blowing a thin blouse gently against a sore nipple sends a pain down to your toes: 'My heart sank every time the baby woke up because that meant another feed.' But even sore, cracked or bleeding nipples will heal very quickly if you get the right help. The priority is to position the baby well at the breast so that the nipple area is well inside, away from friction. Neither breastmilk nor the baby's saliva will damage your nipple, so the baby can be kept at the breast if the position is improved. Blood from cracks does not harm the baby. Alternatively, another suggestion you may be given is to rest the nipple. But this means you must allow milk to build up uncomfortably, or use a pump which may be even more painful although you can control the suction.

If sore nipples are a problem, it can help to let the baby suck first on the less sore side while she is eager to get milk flowing and to return her to this one for her less careful comfort feeding at the end of the feed.

Do get skilled help for pain. In nearly the best possible situations it can happen, but it can be helped.

Nipple shields

There is no doubt that some mothers have found nipple shields useful, but they have their own difficulties. They cut down the flow of milk because your breast is not being stimulated directly and babies can get addicted to the use of shields.

If you do use a nipple shield and the baby refuses to feed without one, try turning it inside out and cutting it away a bit at a time from the centre where the holes are, watching for sharp edges.

'*I tried various ploys over five weeks to wean him from the shield but they just turned feeding times into a battleground . . . I was overflowing with milk and he was a very strong sucker but over the five weeks his feeding times got closer and closer till he was wanting to feed every two hours.*'

Nipples in all shapes and sizes

If you are worried about the shape of one or both of your nipples, you need to know that most enthusiastic breastfeeding babies will take any shape of nipple and breast and form a long soft 'teat' which suits them. If necessary, it may help to pull out the nipple as much as possible by using a breastpump before feeds. One side may be easier for the baby to get on to than the other, and it is quite possible to feed a baby from one side (think of the mothers of twins) and express milk from the side which the baby finds more difficult. Some babies will move back on to this breast after a while, once their mouths are bigger and they have grown more skilled in breastfeeding.

Engorgement

This does go away of its own accord, but it can be pretty unpleasant, especially if you are not able to feed the baby as often as you had hoped to during the day or so when your breasts are swollen. The main worry with engorgement is that because the tissue behind the areola is so full of fluid, it is hard and shiny, making it difficult for the baby to get a grip on the breast tissue without hurting you and sliding forwards towards just the nipple. Various things may help.

- gently – very gently – massage your breasts from the edges towards the nipple
- encourage milk to flow by sitting in a warm bath and either submerging your breasts or douching them with warm water, or apply warm face flannels

- use your fingers to slowly press back the swelling from all the way around the areola so that the baby can get a softer mouthful of breast tissue
- use cold face flannels *after* feeds in order to calm the breast down and to help reduce the swelling
- insert green cabbage leaves between your bra and your breast – this really does seem to work

If you are really full, ask if you may use an electric-pump once or twice to remove every drop of milk available at that time. Normally, taking out lots of milk tells the body to make more, but this does seem to relieve engorgement at this stage. You can also ask the midwife for painkillers.

Helping sore nipples to heal

Mothers have found these things useful to try:
- keeping nipples dry, with no soggy breast pads
- letting fresh air to them, and if available, a little sunlight
- sleeping naked under cotton sheets (on towels if you leak)
- encouraging the milk to flow before the baby begins to feed by warming your breasts, perhaps with a face flannel
- massaging milk down from the far parts of the breast
- stopping using any cream or spray – in case of sensitivity to it
- changing the position of the baby around the breast
- applying pure lanolin ointment to any crack (unless you are allergic to wool)

These things are useful to avoid:
- letting the baby suck in a 'lost' breast when she has let go
- dragging the baby's mouth off the breast

Lots of milk?

If, when your milk comes in, the baby seems very quickly overwhelmed, let her come off and then you can catch the surplus gushes in a nappy. She may just lie there as milk comes down for her and forget the hard work needed, and so you may have to teach her again how to open her mouth and so on.

Calming a panicky baby

Some babies panic very quickly and seem to struggle at the breast, their heads bobbing from side to side in an exaggerated search for the breast, even though it is there all the time, probably dripping with milk: 'she was so anxious to feed that she would throw herself around in frustration and find it difficult to latch on.' Mothers sometimes feel as if their babies are 'fighting' them, which is upsetting. It can be worth gently rousing a baby like this before she is hungry and taking time to talk to her, unwrap her, and let her skin and yours touch in a reassuring way, before offering her the breast while she is alert but not screaming. While they are still asleep or half-awake, some babies will actually open their mouths wide if their lips are gently brushed. It may also help to hold the baby in a different position from that which she is used to in feeding, and many mothers find they are instinctively repeating that the milk is there all the time, nice and ready for her. This may calm you both. It can be a temptation to sit with your teeth gritted in total silence. Getting the milk flowing, with warmth, massage and a little milk gently expressed into her mouth first may be reassuring.

Back to positioning

Several pointers may show that the baby is not as well positioned as she needs to be. For example, a baby who is feeding every hour, all day and night, or who is feeding for say an hour and a half every time may need help to learn how to feed well. Or, if what is in the nappy is still 'tarry' after the third or fourth day (despite your being able to feed your baby in an unrestricted way), you may need to make sure that the baby is receiving enough milk, and that means again looking at her position on the breast. It is worth checking that you are not holding her too far away from the breast towards the side of your body as if you were going to pop the breast in like a bottle. Be sure too that the baby does not have her chin down on her chest, which makes it difficult to swallow. She should be in a fairly straight line, not curled round like a shrimp. This is often easier on one side than the other (for most mothers it seems to be the right that brings more problems). Try having a look at what you do easily on the 'good' side and thinking how to make a mirror image of this on the other side. Look back at the previous pages on positioning and attaching the baby and get help if you need it. It is rarely too late for this.

Clicking noises during feeds also suggest this may be less than perfect. You are hoping for an initial short burst of suckling and then deep jawings and swallowings. If the fast sucking goes on all the way through the feed, again ask for help and check the positioning (see pages 25–34).

Once a baby is well fixed, her attention tends to be on feeding: suckling and swallowing takes a lot of concentration and effort, and her arms should stop waving about. If they do not and she is restless, then there may well be a problem with how she is attached to the breast.

If you feel the baby goes on right, and then tends to slide off, look again at whether she is properly supported: she should not have to hang on. If she begins to hurt you, it is a good move to break the suction with your little finger and start again. If things do not seem to improve, it is a good idea to find someone who has experience of observing breastfeeding and who can help by watching as you feed. Ask her to talk you through any changes she feels may help.

Sleepy babies

If she starts to fall asleep as soon as the nipple and breast are in her mouth this could again be because she is not as well attached to the breast as she might be. Or she may still be sleepy from painkilling drugs you received in labour, or treatment after a caesarean. It may help to unwrap her, and wipe her face gently with a cool cloth. Making gentle circles on the skin of the instep of your baby's foot often wakes her up or keeps her awake to feed. If you decide to wake her, it is more likely she will come round if she is already stirring. Watch for her moving in her sleep and making noises. She may be able to have her interest kept up by changing sides as soon as her suckling slows down, making many let-downs. She will get lots of foremilk this way, but may take more than if she just went to sleep on the first side before she got to the creamier milk. You can squeeze milk into her mouth to encourage her to learn to swallow even if she is half asleep and so make energy to be able to feed later. This helps to avoid a vicious circle where the baby is sleepy and so can't feed and so on. Lifting her jaw up gently may stimulate her to continue suckling.

Common medical concerns

Jaundice

Jaundice is a common condition in small babies, and is more likely with premature births. It is only a temporary problem. Jaundice is a symptom, like a rash, not a disease. Most of the babies who develop it after a few days, and begin to look sun-tanned as a consequence, have normal or 'physiological' jaundice. This is caused when a yellow pigment called bilirubin is not processed fast enough from their bodies by their livers. It is usually gone within a week or so.

If the jaundice seems to be more than just mild, the bilirubin level of the baby is tested by a small blood sample and sometimes no treatment is necessary. If it is, then the baby, wearing a mask or with a perspex cover above her head to protect her eyes, is put under lights which imitate sunlight and help to break down the pigment so that the liver can get rid of it faster.

You can help by feeding the baby as much as she wants, aiming to allow her to reach some hindmilk. Research has shown that breastmilk itself – with its speedy passage through the gut – helps your baby to pass bilirubin into her nappy with her motions (rather than reabsorbing it). It used to be thought that bilirubin could somehow be washed out with water like a dye; this is not the case, but your colostrum and milk will do the job well.*

Unfortunately, sometimes both jaundice and the treatment make babies sleepy, leaving mothers feeling uncomfortable, and the babies not keen to learn active breastfeeding. You can try the suggestions for waking sleepy babies offered on page 56, and if the baby is under the lights, ask whether it is possible to have her out to unwrap and hold before you try to feed. The treatment causes more and looser motions to get rid of the bilirubin, so the baby may be thirsty. If it is suggested that the baby needs water in addition to your milk this could be given on a spoon to avoid her being confused by a teat. Your milk is roughly 90 per cent water anyway.

As jaundice is only a symptom, medical staff will monitor the situation in case there is a different cause, such as illness in the baby. There is another kind of jaundice, called 'breastfeeding jaundice' which produces similar symptoms but does not usually begin until several days after the normal kind. It is caused by a reaction in the baby to something in her mother's milk. Again, this is not a worrying condition, although it may take longer to fade. Doctors used to suggest interrupting breastfeeding to test whether this was what the problem was, but usually now other tests can be done to make sure there is no other more serious cause.

After a caesarean

It is you who have the problems here: 'The combination of a drip in the back of my hand, very sore tummy, heavy baby and being confined to bed did not make for easy cuddling, let alone anything else.' It may be 24 hours before you can slowly get out of bed, and before that you will probably be on a drip, feeding you intravenously, with a slow return to real food after that. You and your baby both have good food stores laid down in pregnancy so although you may not have eaten for some time, and are on a drip for a while, your milk will still arrive and be fine for the baby.

If you have had an epidural or spinal anaesthetic you will have little pain straight after birth, and be quite alert so this can be a good time to try the first feed. However, there is no rush.

Delivery beds are not ideal places to breastfeed, so you may need to experiment to find comfortable positions, with pillows, and lots of help: 'I wasn't shown any special positions for holding her for feeding, so I just laid her across my tummy, the most painful position of all.' If you have had a general anaesthetic you may be propped up to keep your lungs clear, so you need help with pillows to be able to feed in a good position without pulling the breast out of the baby's mouth. You will probably need a small pillow or cot blanket to stop the baby from kicking your sore scar area. The underarm position, sometimes called the 'football' hold, can be useful, and lying down is a possibility. Pull the whole baby towards you as you position her at the breast, and hold her close to your chest to turn over. A pillow under your ribs can be useful to move you up in relation to her if if necessary, or you can put a pillow between your head and an upstretched arm to stop it 'going to sleep'.

'Because of the epidural and the caesarean, I could not at first sit up straight enough to see what was happening when latching on was taking place and while the baby was feeding. It was difficult for me to tell whether she was positioned correctly or not.'

Nursing staff realise that after caesareans you need more assistance, so do not be afraid to ask for help in picking up and positioning your baby. It may feel more difficult if you are in a single room but ring the bell: staff would rather help you early to independence.

As colostrum arrives in small quantities there is usually no concern about sleeping pills or painkillers affecting the baby much. The National Childbirth Trust produces a leaflet about feeding a baby after a section. Mothers' reactions to having had a caesarean varies, depending on all kinds of factors such as the surprise element involved. Women describe feeling shocked or guilty, finding difficulty in feeling the baby is theirs, or relief at having been rescued from an impossible situation. Breastfeeding can seem very important: 'I needed to feel I could succeed at something, having "failed" at a normal delivery.'

Low blood sugar levels in babies

This condition, also referred to as hypoglycaemia, is a relatively recent concern for medical staff and parents. It is now realised that it is possible for some babies to run out of energy – or 'fuel' – and become ill as a result, possibly developing conditions which affect their long-term brain development. Many of the babies who receive bottles or cups of formula in hospital are thought to have, or to be at risk of developing, low blood sugar levels. However, it is clear from recent authoritative guidelines that healthy babies born around the time they were expected need neither testing nor extra fluid.* Such babies are able to use other fuels in their own body. Beginning breastfeeding when the baby is ready after birth and keeping her close with skin to skin contact are very good ways to help her stay warm and give her energy from the start so that it is less likely that she will have a problem with blood sugar levels.

Hypoglycaemia is more likely where a baby is ill, born prematurely or has a mother with diabetes, and so the blood of these babies may be routinely tested for sugar levels. There are various ways of doing this. One of the most frequently used tests involves taking a tiny amount of blood from the baby's heel and testing it with a 'BM stix' or 'dextrostix'. However, these 'stix' are not designed for use with babies, and more accurate readings are given by other methods of testing. Currently there is also a variety of medical opinions about the level of blood sugar which is acceptable, the criteria for testing a baby (such as the length of time between the baby wanting to be fed) and the action to be taken. In most hospitals formula is not offered until the mother has agreed to this happening, so you will be able to think about what is suggested. If you are told that your baby needs a formula feed, you may like to ask about the reasons and be sure that an accurate blood sugar level has been obtained.

The level at which babies are deemed to need rapid extra food varies according to the interpretation of the research by consultant paediatricians. For a mother wishing to breastfeed, the difficulty is that in some hospitals staff may be quick to suggest that babies need either dextrose (a sugar and water solution) or formula to raise their blood sugar level. In one hospital it may be that the paediatrician who finds a baby with a low blood sugar level suggests that another test is done after a breastfeed, while in another a bottle of formula is offered immediately. As it is especially the long sleeps after birth which cause concern – whether or not the baby has fed from the mother – it may be useful to look at ideas for waking up sleepy babies (see page 56) or to ask the midwife to help you get the baby breastfeeding before a bottle is suggested. The lengths of time between feeds that hospitals may be happy about vary between four and eight hours. These long sleeps are more likely after pethidine has been given for pain in labour. The antidote to pethidine, narcan, does not work for as long as pethidine. If your baby is sleepy, it could be useful to ask for a further dose to help her feel less drowsy. If holding the baby skin to skin was not possible after birth or was cut short, doing this again and allowing your baby to come round and find your breast for herself may be the best way of stimulating her to feed. Being together in a bath (the right temperature for the baby of course) can also be helpful.

When faced with possible medical repercussions, or having to offer a bottle which may not be what you had planned, it is hard to remain calm. You might be able to persuade staff to let you feed the baby first, with breastmilk, (the food most easily and quickly absorbed by the baby), before another test to see if a complementary feed or fluid needs to be given. A small amount of colostrum can help and may be given in a cup if the basic problem is that the baby is not yet breastfeeding. If this is because she is sleepy, it is worth trying the ideas for waking a baby and keeping her feeding suggested on page 56 and looking at the section on page 30 about interesting the baby in the breast. You might also ask whether formula could be offered by means other than a bottle or find out whether breastmilk is available, as there are still a few hospitals with milk banks. Hypoglycaemia is a quickly passing phase and in the long term should not damage your chances of breastfeeding: 'In hospital Oliver had some supplementary bottles of formula because his blood sugar level was low . . . but he always had breast first and once my milk arrived he refused formula.'

Twins and more

Having more than one baby is obviously a lot more work from the beginning. Some mothers say they have found it hard to fall in love with two or more babies at once. You are also more likely to have a caesarean section, and also to have premature babies. It can be useful therefore to have looked at the section on expressing milk (pages 156–159). On the other hand, engorgement may be less of a problem.

> *'I did once feed one twin twice and*
> *left the other one!'*

You will obviously need a good deal of physical assistance during your time in hospital. If you are able to feed the babies right away, getting the position right is important as you will get more wear on each nipple if it is not safely in the soft back of the babies' mouths.

> *'I found that one breast seemed to produce more*
> *milk than the other, perhaps because it was easier to*
> *"milk". (I) thought it might be the baby's technique*
> *but found by trial and error that this was not so. As a*
> *result I fed each baby exclusively from his "own"*
> *breast for one week then swapped them over the*
> *next – their weight gain usually showed about*
> *4oz difference each week.'*

Even if the twins are identical – biologically, and to everyone else – you may find they feed slightly differently. Some mothers feel that feeding the babies together is the answer to the difficulty of finding time to feed twice as much. This maybe helpful to the levels of the milk-making hormone, which needs to be higher, of course, in the mother of multiples. If one baby is less good at suckling the other can keep up the milk supply and it may help to feed two together when you have got the hang of it to help let-down for the one who is less sure. The babies can both be held underarm, both across your lap or with a mixture of the two. If there are three, you need obviously to think about feeding in rotation, getting help with holding and feeding and perhaps using a bottle sometimes with your own or formula milk. One mother described feeding more than one baby as, 'supply and demand theory stretched to the limit – not really possible to feed more frequently than all the time!'

Other mothers find it better to teach the babies one at a time about getting on to the breast well, and that this gives them a chance to get to know their babies individually too. If the baby who is being kept waiting is crying, this may distress you while you feed the other one, and it may be that someone else could try to calm her while you feed.

Some mothers keep a breast for each baby, as their requirements, especially if they are just siblings who arrived together, may be quite different. Others deliberately change breasts each time to keep their own supply balanced.

Very special babies

If your baby or babies are in the Special Care Baby Unit, you have the extra difficulty of feeding them indirectly via a breast-pump. Chapter 12 includes information about premature babies. Chapter 11 has extra details about expressing. Support organisations and leaflets are listed at the back of the book.

When there is any problem with a baby or a mother there can sometimes be a tendency for people to assume that breastfeeding is impossible and that it is not important compared with the solving of a medical concern. In fact breastfeeding is more important than ever if a baby is ill. It may be very difficult but is rarely impossible. Even if it has had to stop for a while, it is possible to begin again (see Relactation, page 175). It is important to feel, both at the time and later, that you were able to get access to the information you needed to see all the options in any special situation. Any approach other than 'just breastfeeding' may help but may also hinder what you want to do long-term. For example, the use of teats, dummies, nipple shields and so on may occasionally be useful but can equally lead to the end of breast-feeding. For instance, it is not easy to tell which babies will find teats very rewarding (although babies who have not yet experienced a really satisfying breastfeed are probably going to find that having the milk available right away is a relief). It is always worth considering the benefits and risks of any intervention and looking at alternatives or whether doing nothing might be better. You may find it helpful to negotiate for some time and further explanation as you make up your mind.

CHAPTER FIVE

Getting and using help

---

*'The staff at the hospital were marvellous, very patient
and understanding. Many of the other first-time mums
on my ward were also experiencing problems and
many a sleepless night in the nursery was spent with us
all trying to get our babies to latch on!'*

It is likely that you will be helped in all kinds of ways by people
you do not know during the immediate post-natal period, unless
you number among the 2 per cent of women who have their
babies at home. You will be shown, for example, how to put
your baby to sleep on her back, as latest research suggests this is
the safest position until she is old enough to choose for herself by
rolling over.

At other times, and in other places, the person helping to
establish breastfeeding was not, and is not, trained to do this,
but simply knows the mother well, offers meals, tips, experience
and the assumption that it will work. This is unusual now but it
nevertheless can happen: 'I was lucky to have a good friend in
the next bed who was on to her third baby and was an absolute
fount of useful advice, tips and help (even at 2am).'

Most hospital policies and midwives try to recognise that
you and your baby are individuals, and they are ready to be flexible. For example, one mother relates that, 'For some unknown
reason he would not latch on to my right breast. I was advised by
the midwife in the hospital to hold him under my arm with his
legs behind me.'

Health professionals are used to helping; that is partly why they chose to do what they are doing, but you may not be used to being helped, and find it hard to deal with the personal attention, or to ask for what you need. It can upset you to feel you are asking for more than others. It may be simply that your need is greater, either for physical assistance or for reassurance. Needing help, whether it is asking for a bedpan, or to be shown the best way to hold a baby after a caesarean can make us feel vulnerable, but breastfeeding does need support and midwives are interested in being involved at its beginning.

'I still could not get in and out of my chair with a baby in my arms, but did not feel guilty that I had to ring for someone . . . I accepted that it would be better for all of us if I had help in these early days when we needed it.'

Many mothers feel that they should be able to manage, if the feeding is supposed to be 'natural' and that they have already been rather disruptive by having a baby at all. It is worth remembering how little information we, both mother and baby, enter this new world with. 'I now realise that I was completely unprepared for breastfeeding, just as I was for the first few weeks with my first baby. I am a medical doctor which doesn't help much, but at least I was somewhat informed.'

Trust and good communication, with agreement on the goals of the mother between her and staff, lead to confident starts: 'The staff knew I wanted to breastfeed, but I just couldn't manage it that evening, so we started the next day.'

Help – everyone
says something different

Your family and friends may visit, each bringing their own set of ideas and recommendations for feeding, while they hope you are open to suggestions. It can be a good idea to take all they say and wait until later to decide which information or experiences are useful for you and your baby. You can also choose from different ideas in leaflets or books, deciding which best fits you and your baby. Always bear in mind, though, that what works one time may not work another.

Most of your interaction, however, will be with the health professionals who are caring for you. They too come from different families and wider backgrounds, and mixed in with information about feeding will be their own attitudes towards it, just as it is for your family and friends. They will have been trained by lots of different people with varying ideas for practical help. Most midwives feel that there is ample evidence that breastmilk is the best food for young babies, but may be reluctant to seem to be 'pushing' breastfeeding, in case a bottle-feeding mother might feel guilty about this. They may also feel, having seen such a lot of the first rather fraught few days, and little of the comparatively calm journey ahead, that it all looks like a lot of bother for only a little reward.

You may hear a variety of answers to questions you ask, and be shown several 'right' ways to do things. Each way of putting it may be leading to the same thing, or you may be up against conflicting opinions: 'Different midwives give different advice leaving you floundering as to what to do for the best.' It can feel hard to know who to trust – you could just try each idea in turn and see which works, and try to keep calm. You could explain each time what the previous suggestion was and ask if the two ideas are compatible.

Research points to a consistent approach being helpful to the breastfeeding mother. Sadly, this is hard for hospitals to achieve, with rotas for staff and short stays for mothers, as well as the rapid changes in the stages of breastfeeding, particularly during the first week: 'Some advised feeding in bed, others reprimanded me for cuddling him on the bed as it was "dangerous".'

It has been suggested that it is not a good idea to keep asking everyone who comes into the ward for their advice about feeding, but to stick to one or two people who you trust. This sounds sensible, but you may find that a person who you feel is a good listener and skilled at helping you to position the baby, will not be back on duty again until after you have gone home: 'One midwife got him latched on well with me lying down. She then went off duty, never to be seen again.'

Helping yourself

'On the second day, he was starving, and of course my milk hadn't come in. He just screamed from about midnight till three in the morning, and although he was sucking very regularly he was obviously very upset. I was starting to panic so I wheeled his cot into the nursery and thought I might give him a bottle. He was definitely not impressed by distilled water . . . what saved me from the crisis was my secret store of rescue food. My husband had brought me some date slice which I had made before I came into hospital. I climbed back into bed, wolfed down a couple of slices, took Daniel into bed with me and tried sticking him on again. (I kept thinking "get a grip, Kate, everything's going to be OK!") This time, although there was still no milk, the sucking seemed to calm him down. We settled down into a long sleep together and woke up again feeling a lot better at about 8am.'

Like this mother, it is wise to look at ways of helping yourself and perhaps of asking for help even if you feel more like pretending there is not a problem. Some women simply wait until they are home to sort things out, even choosing to bottle-feed briefly in hospital before putting the baby back on the breast. This seems a shame as it may risk interfering with the baby's learning about suckling. There may be allergies in your family which make you feel it is especially important that nothing but breastmilk is given to your baby.

You can, of course, help yourself in all kinds of ways, like using any relaxation you have learnt if you feel fraught. Understanding the basic points about how breastfeeding works, and particularly how to get the baby to take the breast well, will be useful. This means that you will then understand which practices go with the way that research shows breastfeeding works, rather than the ways in which we know it can be made harder for mothers. However, you may have learnt from dealings with health professionals in the past that knowing something is regarded sometimes with some suspicion, so it can help to frame your points carefully. For example, if you are being told to limit the time of the baby at the breast if your nipples are sore you could ask for an explanation of why this suggestion may help as you have understood that this is no longer felt to be helpful. You can also ask for someone to watch the next feed to make sure you are getting the baby attached in a way that will not hurt you.

Time with the baby in simply skin-to-skin touching, and getting to know each other will help with difficult breastfeeding. Warm hospital wards are a good place for this:

'The following day my husband brought in *Breast is Best*, and I become filled with resolve. My milk was coming in and I was fed up trying to please everyone else. I decided that my baby must be my priority and on reading that book anew I realised that yes, I was capable of breastfeeding, and no, he didn't need water or formula milk. I closed the floral curtains, took off the baby's various blankets and spent hours holding him, letting him gradually wake up . . . he eventually did latch on and started to suck . . . we had worked out breastfeeding together. I was very aware of the relationship being so different from what I had expected before the birth. We had both been novices and both needed each other's help.'

Saying what you mean

Being a patient is not easy. It may be difficult to say how you feel about the way you had intended to feed the baby. It can feel sometimes as if the main aim in hospital is not to be a nuisance, particularly when they have just created yet another patient. Being determined about breastfeeding can almost feel like selfishness: kindly, or cross, pressure to eat meals instead of feeding may be teaching you to ignore your baby's cry which is meant to be hard to do. It is difficult to please everyone at once, and yet this is a vulnerable time. Perhaps your partner's support, in person or not, may make it easier to say 'we have decided that we would like to make sure the baby's needs come first', or whatever you feel is important.

One of the ways which can be helpful in communicating your needs clearly to your helpers is to use some of the techniques of assertiveness. This does not mean you have to be aggressive or loudly insistent. It is basically a way of being honest as you make your point, rather than apologetic or angry. One such technique is the 'broken record' where you acknowledge the other person's point calmly, but also restate your own point of view. An example might be: 'I can see you feel it would be a bad idea to let the baby feed so long at a time, but my nipples are not sore, and we all feel the position is right so I would like to continue.'

Who is who?

'Each time I wanted to try to feed the baby I had to go to the desk and ask for help. I asked everyone wearing a uniform (having never been in hospital before I didn't know that a sister was senior to a staff midwife, and that grey uniforms were worn by people who weren't midwives at all. Just auxiliaries – but who seemed willing to give advice too.)"

It may not be easy to know who is the most likely person to be right, even at the simple level of knowing how much training a health professional has. In some hospitals, only midwives are allowed to offer advice, but it must be very hard when confronted by a distressed mother not to say something, even if you are not supposed to. It might be a good idea to find out what uniforms each kind of member of staff wear – this varies from hospital to hospital. As breastfeeding is not a medical area, but a biological, social, and psychological one, any staff, including an auxiliary who has fed three children with pleasure and knows how to cheer you up, may do you more good than someone else who is suspicious of the way the whole thing works. But others may be insufficiently informed: 'When my daughter was about 24 hours old I asked if I could use the breast pump and feed my baby with expressed milk. The nurse (an SEN) who I talked to said, "There's no point – your milk hasn't come in yet." Fortunately, through NCT classes, I had heard of colostrum, and I insisted.'

In some hospitals, midwives with a particular interest in breastfeeding may have a special role. You may find there are 'lactation sisters', or similarly titled staff, at the hospital during the day, whom other staff may suggest you talk to. In a few

Helping to improve breastfeeding

It might help to:

- wear nursing bras that do not dig in to your breast, with plenty of room for adjustment during engorgement
- use breast pads without waterproof backing if you leak (soggy pads can lead to soreness). Pads with 'one-way tissue' are fine
- pack change to phone out of the hospital to your supporter, a breastfeeding counsellor, etc
- wear comfortable night clothes for feeding in
- use a pillow or folded blanket to support the baby at the most comfortable height
- use face cloths for either warming your breasts, or for cooling them and the baby
- drink liquids when you need to
- write down reminders of important points – your own or taken from a familiar book

Less helpful things are:

- creams – they trap moisture. If you feel you must use them, try any on the inside of your elbow first. Applying lanolin to any cracks (avoiding uncracked skin) may help to prevent them from opening up. Remember, though, that if you are sore, your first priority is to get good help with positioning
- sprays – they discourage bacteria but bacteria are friendly. For example, they can destroy thrush
- nipple shields – use them if it is suggested that the only alternative is to rest for a couple of days. They cut down milk supply so you need to offer longer feeds. Once your milk has arrived, you could use them to get the baby going, then take them off for the rest of the feed
- bras with 'trap door' openings, which dig into your breast and can cause a 'traffic jam' making a blocked duct more likely

continued

- 'drip catchers' – like a little plate with a hole and a bowl fixed together to catch milk from one side. They can press and cause blocked ducts, and they stimulate more milk; however, they are OK for catching milk on one side while you feed on the other
- there is a good argument for using very little 'helpful' equipment unless you are sure you need it.

hospitals, National Childbirth Trust breastfeeding counsellors visit the ward to help mothers, working alongside midwifery staff. Of course, anyone can ring out to speak to a counsellor, who will try to help and may be able to offer a visit.

'The midwife had breastfed her own baby after a caesarean, so not only knew such a feat was possible, but knew some of the necessary tricks.'

Young staff may be more recently trained and well informed, especially if they happen to have taken a special interest in breastfeeding. Older staff may have had a great deal of experience which has taught them how to be of help. One may have tried to breastfeed, found it very hard, and be quick to try to 'rescue' you. Older staff may have found it easier to suggest bottles and find demand feeding disruptive to the ward routine. 'I feel that following your instincts is very important. But also confidence in doing so is essential and that even as a health visitor for some six years I did not find it very easy to hold on to. Pressures to give up, however subtle and unwitting, from relatives and staff (especially kind ones!!) are very powerful.'

You are not in a position to 'interview' everyone who offers a suggestion to see where they are 'coming from', but it may help to ask a general question about mothers' problems. If the answer is something like, 'Yes, breastfeeding is not really all that easy, and the modern milks are very good' or, 'Some people do have problems at first but it seems worth it in the end', you may be able to decide on the helper's attitude.

It is worth remembering that if you were at home, the ideas you would be receiving would be more likely to feel like suggestions. You might then be more free to try them and not continue with them if they seemed unhelpful. In hospital, because it feels more as if you will be observed, one idea can be to try to look quite determined and so seem not to be in need of any help. Saying 'It's fine', though, when you think it isn't, will not necessarily help. It may be better to listen to suggestions, even if this means you may feel you need to say that you would rather not do what has been suggested. It is a good idea here to ask whether there are any alternatives to the suggestion made, explaining that you would prefer not to do something which you feel might be unhelpful in the long term. It may, however, be that what you see as a worrying idea is only being suggested for a short time and is considered medically necessary. An area in which this may happen would be if the baby were considered to have low blood sugar (see page 59). Whatever the cause, you are entitled to a proper explanation so persist in getting it.

Many other people also come on to a ward – other patients, clerks, porters, social workers, window cleaners and nursery nurses. Their opinions on your baby crying or 'feeding again', may also be offered, and need filtering in the light of your understanding. You may also see some doctors as they do their rounds, sometimes in suits or dresses, or white coats. Obstetricians have some interest in breastfeeding and may have comments to make. Paediatricians, baby specialists, work with ill and premature babies.

Asking for help

Whole groups of people may be considered as a good bet for breastfeeding success or failure, because they belong to a certain group. For example, professional women are sometimes seen as being in danger of having a lot of problems because they will be 'neurotic' about feeding. Black women may be seen as having few problems and so needing no help. Doctors' wives, nurses, and midwives similarly say that they are often left to feed alone: 'Being a nurse myself I was left to my own devices. The feeling from many of the ward staff was that I "should know what to do." I didn't!' If you feel you need help, you may need to seek it clearly.

Experienced mothers, even if they have breastfed successfully, still may need reminding of how to position the newborn baby – something which is quite different from the way in which you let a one-year-old take the breast: 'He was very difficult to start to feed and this time I didn't get much help from midwives. Second-time mums are supposed to find it easy.' If you did not breastfeed last time or found it difficult, tell the staff.

Time

Time spent with someone in need is so much appreciated by all of us and this is especially true of new mothers. This mother had a baby who had been in Special Care and so needed extra help to get used to breastfeeding: 'a wonderful midwife spent some time with me persuading Duncan to latch on. With her help, and quite a bit of patience, I managed to introduce him to the breast.'

A hospital midwife is often now desperately short of time, with up to 30 or more mothers to care for alone, and the Royal College of Midwives' book itself regrets that she may only have one or two opportunities to help each mother: 'Sometimes I was promised help but the midwife was called to a crisis in a different room and forgot to come later.' Some midwives may sometimes feel it is a really useful shortcut to take your breast and the baby and put them together, but an experienced and wise midwife knows it is better to work first at you learning for yourself what to do, so that you feel more confident about doing it over and over again. If your midwife helps you by moving your baby and breast together, but says little, it is well worth asking her to describe what she is doing so that you can understand how to repeat this later. Experienced midwives seem now often to be feeling that the best thing is to talk mothers through positioning with as little physical assistance as possible. She is not carrying out a clinical procedure which only happens once or twice, but teaching you and your baby to become efficiently attached to one another, so that milk can be available for months to come. She may forget to tell you what is important about the way she is doing this, simply because she is concentrating hard on the baby's position. Next time you may be managing on your own, without expert help.

Help you may not enjoy

Staff may feel much freer to handle your breasts than you are comfortable with. If they warn you, 'let's just tickle his mouth with your nipple, all right?' before the touch you this may be OK, or you can say 'I'd like to try myself.' Your midwife may wish to express a little milk to show you it is there, and to remind the baby of what is good about breastfeeding, especially if she is sleepy or panic-stricken. A midwife may put your breast and the baby's mouth together, to give you an idea of the timing and the feel of good positioning. If she is experienced and gentle this can be helpful. Sometimes, mothers say they feel they were initially being rather too tentative in their movement of the baby to the breast, and ask for this kind of help. Other mothers do not like being handled and would prefer to try for themselves.

One way suggested by health professionals is for the midwife to put her hands over yours and just help you to time the crucial moment of the 'approach' of the baby, when her mouth is wide open. You could ask your midwife to do this for you. She may, however, say that she would rather not work in this way if she has not had the experience in which case she may be able to find someone else.

If you find being handled painful or upsetting, you need to say so and again ask why it is being done, and whether you could do it yourself. If it is done roughly it can result in bruising in the mother's breast. Mothers do not find it helpful to have the skin of the areola puckered and the nipple squeezed into the baby's mouth, while the back of her head is held in place. This can lead to some babies' becoming very resistant to feeding.

'I became more and more frustrated as I couldn't get her on properly. The staff help that night consisted of taking my breast in one hand, her head in the other and ramming them together until a contact was made! By morning I'd decided to bottle-feed.'

Strategies for managing after unkind or unhelpful remarks

'The sister arrived, took one look and announced to everyone "You'll never breastfeed with nipples like those, I should give up before you get sore and give him a bottle." I felt like she'd have hurt me less if she'd slapped me in the face. However, I was determined I wasn't going to give up without a fight and I plucked up courage and asked for help to try and latch him on. The sister had no time for silly mums who didn't know what was best for their babies and sent a student midwife who was lovely and sat with me for over an hour.'

The second time, this mother was more prepared. 'Back on the postnatal ward I had a battle to prevent the staff taking Claire away to give her a bottle (You've got no milk yet, she's big and hungry, etcetera, etcetera). I was on the phone to the breast-feeding counsellor twice in the first 24 hours. She gave me the strength to keep saying no.'

Hurtful and demoralising remarks by others, whether health professionals, relations or friends, do not always offer medical or nursing facts but can be unsought opinions based on preju-dice. Remarks about 'naughty', 'greedy', 'demanding' babies, and so on, may feel quite upsetting. You can always explain this, saying how you feel: 'When you keep calling my baby an awk-ward customer, it does upset me.'

For a confident, second-time around mother, though, com-ments such as these may drop like water off a duck's back.

'Much to the scorn of the midwife I put my second son straight to the breast after his birth.'

Other actions or feelings arise from trying to protect the mother from the baby's demands. For example, here is an extract from the diary of a second-time breastfeeder: 'Day 4: During the night Emily was awake every two hours for a feed, and we slept in between. I never saw a member of the night-staff but they were aware that I was up, because the day staff kept comment-ing on my "bad night", and I kept insisting it wasn't . . . I feel they don't appreciate that the frequent feeds are necessary to stimulate my milk supply. I am very pleased that I am in a single cubicle.'

'Day 5: All that frequent feeding has worked. Emily settled about 10pm and woke around 1am and 5am for a feed.'

To help improve situations such as these, it would be good if mothers could also be very clear about which actions and words *did* help them as they thanked their carers.

More decisions

Of course, advice may be absolutely right, and you may realise this in the light of day. Wherever possible, it can be useful to give yourself time to think about how it all fits together. If there is a decision to make, many mothers would find it easier to ask for time to talk it over with their supporters if they are still there, or to wait until visiting time, or to make a phone call if the visitors have gone. Write all the suggestions down if you feel this will help you to prioritise them. A helper who says feeding the baby will make a 'rod for your own back' is simply repeating something which has no relevance to research. One who is concerned that very frequent feeding means the position may need to be improved and asks if you would like her to watch you feed, is offering you something very useful. You may find it valuable to try to find out why those offering what seems unhelpful advice feel as they do. If you encourage a person to talk, you may find there is quite a lot of hurt behind the remark which is to do with *their* experience and very little to do with yours. Understanding this may help to calm you down and also gives the helper a chance to defuse her feelings.

In some cases, you may find that it isn't the individual caregiver who presents you with a dilemma, but the policy of the hospital.

'It was hospital policy to give all "small-for-dates" babies a bottle of formula in the delivery room . . . What could I do? How could I prevent my daughter, who had not been nourished properly within the womb, from receiving nourishment outside the womb? Perhaps I should have waited for an hour or two to see if she would have breastfed then . . . if I had insisted that she should not be bottle-fed she may eventually have become hungry enough to latch on to the breast, but she may also have become more and more weak and sleepy. I didn't want her to become any more undernourished than she was.'

Test-weighing is another difficult area in which it is easy to feel your capacity to feed is being questioned. Weighing after individual feeds is known to be inaccurate and unhelpful to mothers; only measuring intake over a period of 24 hours with very accurate electrical scales might be useful.

A lot of hard work has been done to improve the care of breastfeeding women in our hospitals during the last ten years. This means that the policies and practices of staff should be moving towards a far more consistent and helpful approach. Your honest feedback after a stay in hospital can propel this movement forward.

Going home

Increasingly, even for first-time mothers, in some larger hospitals, you are able to – or encouraged to – go home within a couple of days of the birth if everything is straightforward. You will then be cared for by your community midwife until the baby is at least ten days old, a service uncommon in other countries and now under some threat here. You may feel relief at being home, hopefully with people you know well, where you are able to do things in your own way, and in your own time, but worry that you have lost your instantly available support for new skills such as breastfeeding. You set out, feeling a little alone perhaps, on this new journey.

CHAPTER SIX

At home

'I felt sure that at home in my comfortable low, wide bed, not covered in plastic sheeting, in a cooler temperature, with my husband and little boy (who had never before been separated from me) that breastfeeding would be no problem at all . . . once home Joshua "woke up" to feeding and we both settled down, no problem.'

After hospital, home can seem very welcoming or you may find you feel unsupported, especially at night: 'I thought that at home, in my own environment, breastfeeding would suddenly come right, but it didn't. It was worse because there were no midwives to help.' There will be help, though, even if it is not on tap all the time: 'On the second day a wonderful community midwife came and *watched* me feed (something that never happened in hospital).'

If you have given birth at home you will know that your baby is likely to want to be fed at all sorts of times of the day and night, with possibly several feeds between your normal bedtime and breakfast time. In hospital, sometimes the baby may have been comforted in other ways, so that you only gave one night feed, and she may seem very unsettled at home. She also will have experienced the change from hospital to home, changes in temperature, sounds and activity which may disturb her. If you come home within a couple of days you will still be in the very early, fast-changing period of breastfeeding: 'I was out of hospital in 48 hours and the milk started to come in properly during our first evening at home.'

A new family

For most mothers, who gave birth in hospital, more time is needed in which to rest before picking up fully on the next stage, when they will put together their old life at home with the new task of mothering. This is an opportunity for many to become a 'breastfeeding pair', while also settling the baby into the rest of the family. It is also the first chance for the father to get to know the baby properly. If he is able to look after you and the home for a while you may find this is the ideal solution or others may be called in. If you had a caesarean section, you will need more help at home than the average mother.

Not having to do everything at once, allowing you to recover fully from the birth, labour, and pregnancy is good for all mothers and is not suggested to make sure you 'keep your milk' – it will not be easily put to flight by a brief spell with a vacuum cleaner. It can be a good time to learn to adjust to other people's standards, for your own may change over the next years too.

Back to positioning

It is worth taking time to look again at the position of the baby, especially if you are still sore. Your own furniture may feel more comfortable but can sometimes cause problems, such as having to lean back in a nice soft settee with the baby pulling away from you. One answer is again to have pillows to support you, and the baby if necessary, or you can sit in a straight chair which gives your whole body good support. You will need something under your feet so you have a flat lap to lie the baby on and perhaps a pillow or folded blanket to bring her to just the right height for feeding without you having to hold her or your feet up. Later, as she gets bigger and stronger, you will find she can help herself far more. If you still feel sore it is worth looking back at earlier descriptions and drawings (on pages 27–28). You may find you can more easily attach your baby to the breast if you stand up and then move into a seat, as you will have her held closely to you. Now you are home you may be able to be a bit more experimental with positioning for comfort. If you have had twins, you may find a v-shaped pillow helpful, and you have probably got a sofa to try underarm feeding on. One twins' mother reminded me that it is almost impossible to bottle-feed two babies at the same time, but after some practice it is quite possible with breastfeeding. Mothers using a wheelchair will be more likely to have had a caesarean section and may need to be especially inventive about positioning the baby at the breast. It is not necessarily a solution to lie down, as this could mean a difficult journey in and out of a wheelchair several times a day. One mother with the use of only one hand found that it was hard to get help with this and was disappointed to find herself just as tied up as a bottle-feeding mother at every feed, until she used pillows to support the baby at the breast.

The baby may have more clothes in the way now, and so may you. If may help to get the place warm and go back to feeding with as little between you as possible. Your community midwife will usually be calling during the first ten days of your baby's life. You can remind yourself too, of the basic demand and supply truth of breastfeeding, which means that it still seems to take a large part of the day, and a lot of concentration. It will grow to be easier and it will take a lot less time after a few weeks.

The baby

Your baby should be bright-eyed and alert when awake, not pale and floppy, hot or listless. She will give you a series of signs to show she is interested in feeding. She will begin to search for you, sometimes even as she is coming awake, turning with her mouth opening hopefully, showing you her tongue and, putting her hands to her mouth as she may have done just after birth. You may never hear her crying for food if you are able to keep her with you and watch for these signs. If you have other children it may not be so easy to give exclusive attention every time in this way. You will know that a well baby can cry very loudly but then settle down to feed with relish, the milk glugging down and often making her too full to stay awake. It is not unusual at this stage for a baby to look as if she might sleep for hours and yet sleep only for a few minutes before she wants another little feed. Experienced mothers also know that babies feed much more easily when they are not upset.

Depending on how long you stayed in hospital, the baby's weight may still be going down, or beginning to climb up again. Your community midwife will bring scales to weigh the baby a few times, but they may not quite match those in the hospital so it takes a couple of weighings to get a new base-line. Midwives may be hoping that the baby will average a 25 gram, or 1oz, gain a day in the first 14 days, but mainly they are making sure that there is a steady climb in the weight.

You can expect wetter nappies, still five or six disposables or six to eight terries every day feeling heavy or wet. You can tell what a tablespoonful feels like by pouring in this amount of water into a disposable nappy to test the weight in your hand. This would weigh around an ounce, so you can see that the baby who is weighed naked and who has just wet a nappy, may weigh a few ounces less. Dirty nappies can come once a feed (expect a smallish amount), once a day (expect more), or less frequently (be prepared to bath the baby).

Your baby may well feed eight or more times a day still and will not yet be showing a very obvious pattern of feeds during the day, although there may be hopeful signs of a longer than usual sleep at night, perhaps four or fives hours at a stretch. Often coinciding with the time when your supporter is going home, or returning to work, about ten days after the birth, many babies have their first 'growth spurt', a time of increased feeding, when you do not feel that you can fill them unless you feed much more frequently for longer periods. These 'growth spurts' can happen at any time, and generally the baby takes about 48 hours to persuade your breasts to raise the level of milk manufacture to meet the demand. It can feel like a change of gear, but once the engine has settled down at the new pace, everything will be all right. If you have twins, growth spurts may not be quite synchronised.

When they feel this process happening, many mothers introduce complementary feeds thinking it is a sign that there is *permanently* not enough milk, or feeling that, if there is more time between feeds, their breasts will have time to make more. Extra bottles to 'top up' the baby's feeds in fact work like putting a brick in the lavatory cistern in a drought, stopping more supply from being drawn in. Babies have a strong sucking instinct and will often take a bottle, even if their weight gain shows later that there was no way they really needed it.

Night times

Approaches vary about feeding at night. Your baby will need night feeds for some weeks. To encourage her to learn about how the rest of the family feels about nights and sleeping, avoid talking or playing with her, keep the lights low, and only change her nappy if she is already sore, dirty, or has soaked her clothes so she might become cold. 'Like most mothers I did everything by the book, like putting the light on, feeding and nappy changing in the middle of the night (then wondering why Oliver was wide awake!)'

'Nighttimes, with her sometimes feeding two-hourly after 1am were hard. Sometimes I thought it would be easier to have her completely in bed with us, but my husband wasn't happy with the idea, and I really didn't think I could cope.'

'I usually gave him his night feeds in bed as by feeding him lying down I was often able to doze off and to feel that my sleep hadn't been very interrupted.'

If you are feeding the baby in bed at night, be careful you do not get her too hot with heavy bedclothes, and bear in mind that sleeping pills, alcohol and other drugs may make a parent unaware of her. It is unsafe to have a baby sleeping in your bed if either parent smokes, and sleeping with a baby on a settee can be dangerous. If you have twins, you will be able to think about whether to feed one at once in the night and know you will be woken twice as much; whether to feed one baby and then the other, or to wake them both to feed together when one stirs.

You and breastfeeding

Your milk is increasing in response to the baby's suckling, but during the first week or so after you leave hospital, any engorgement you experienced tends to settle down, so that you are not feeling desperately full all day. However, the baby's needs fluctuate quite a lot in this period, and it seems that your response can be quite extreme, so you can end up waking up very full, or feeling quite flat and empty, especially at the end of the day. Having lots of foremilk in the morning for a thirsty baby is normal, and having less, but creamier and more satisfying hindmilk available in the evening, ready for the night is also normal. It can feel sometimes as if the balance between supply and demand is not quite so well established as it will be, but there is no need to panic. Each feeding period, whether long and meal-like, a quick drink, or a sleepy comfort suckling, will stimulate your body to make more milk available.

If you are still sore all the time, as well as asking for help, you could try all the suggestions made on page 54. A small spray bottle of ice-cold boiled water from the fridge may take the edge off the initial pain. Sore nipples are easily infected by thrush, so if the soreness continues, despite the position being checked carefully, this is worth mentioning to your midwife, health visitor or doctor, in case something could usefully be prescribed for you and the baby.

If you have a lot of milk which spurts or drips from the other breast while you feed, or from the nipple if the baby comes off, then you may feel messy and rather out of control. What can seem reassuring in the first days of feeding can soon turn into a nuisance. This is the time to make sure you are letting the baby decide when to come off the first side, so that she does not get lots of foremilk. If you are offering her a few minutes from each side, your body will keep on making a lot of foremilk for her. You might try splashing your nipples with cold water night and morning to try to exercise the little muscles round the nipple openings which you cannot consciously control.

If your baby seems overwhelmed by the rush of milk, or if she is still upset from being pushed at any time against the breast, you may still need to be calming her, perhaps experimenting with different feeding positions or feeding her before she is hungry, or still half-asleep. If the baby is still sleepy, try feeding her in a room with less light to encourage her to open her eyes, and drop milk beside the nipple when the baby makes an attempt to feed to reward any suckling movement and encourage her to continue.

It may help to know that many women have experienced similar concerns. To find out how they managed, turn to the midwife who is visiting or get in touch with a breastfeeding counsellor.

The baby and you

You will be getting to know your baby quite well now – some wake up urgently hungry, while others lie awake for a while. Breastfeeding may begin to feel more second nature during this first fortnight or so, but for many mothers it takes a lot longer to feel confident, casual and relaxed, so give yourself time. You may begin to know cries of pain, boredom or tiredness from those of hunger, although the breast solves most distress one way or another at this stage, like someone giving us a cup of tea and cake by the fire, and a hug all at the same time. If the crying will not go away, try humming, singing, rocking, using the vacuum cleaner, playing music, or holding the baby against your shoulders or on your lap, tummy between your slightly open legs and patting. If the crying goes on and on, ask for help. It is easy to change to the bottle in desperation, as a big alteration which may make a lot of difference, but there are many other reasons for babies crying.

You

As breastfeeding involves sitting or lying down, it can be seen as a period of rest. You cannot possibly wash up at the same time, for example, but having to get up in the night to a baby at least once really does make you tired. For a mother who already has other difficulties, whether temporary ones such as an infection after the birth, or more longlasting, such as multiple sclerosis, fatigue is an expected side effect, and it is worth remembering that feeding can be seen as a particularly valuable resting time for mothers who are unwell or disabled. Breastfeeding may feel very important too, as it is one thing that you uniquely can do for your baby, while others cook and clean.

Caring for a baby in any way is tiring for all parents, and breastfeeding can feel draining to some women. This can be for all kinds of reasons; for example, someone may have led you to believe it is to be expected. But tiredness is unlikely to have a physical cause connected to breastfeeding, unless you are finding it hard to eat for some reason or are becoming depressed. Making milk is a very efficient process with around 500 calories extra needed overall each day. Some of these are likely to come from the weight you put on in pregnancy and so you need a few extra snacks. Women's biology seems to adjust very efficiently at this time in our lives so that we tick over slightly more slowly. You will probably feel thirstier too, but there is no need to drink a set amount. Just try to notice when you feel hungry or thirsty and do not tell yourself to wait till elevenses or whatever. *You* can demand feed too.

If you have a medical problem such as diabetes you will probably already be in touch with your dietician or specialist. If you are on a specialist diet, it is worth checking that there is no problem. A dietician can be contacted through the GP.

Alcohol affects unborn babies, and experts are cautious about how much is safe for breastfeeding mothers to pass on to their babies. Obviously, it is unwise to take so much that you feel unsafe handling the baby. The odd glass of the wine seems all right but some research has shown that the smell of alcohol is present on the mother's milk, which suggests the taste may well be there too, and babies seem to take less milk after the mother has taken a drink.* Old-fashioned force feeding of stout seems to do very little good, especially if you hate the taste!

Smoking more than 20 cigarettes a day begins to affect the hormones involved in breastfeeding, and 'passive' smoking – being made to breathe in cigarette smoke – is in any case harmful to the baby. So it is important to avoid smoking just before and during breastfeeding and to do it as far away as possible if you cannot stop. As in pregnancy, this is obviously a good time to cut down or stop, but it may be a stressful time when it feels even more necessary. There may be a support group available to help you.

You need to talk about any drugs which are prescribed for pain or to improve any condition with your doctor. If there is a suggestion that a treatment makes breastfeeding impossible, it is worth asking whether any alternative, such as another drug or monitoring the baby for side-effects if possible. If you wish to take some laxatives, as hospital food and birth can make you constipated, avoid ones which work on your whole system, and ask for things which only give you bulk. Some laxatives could be present in the milk and affect the baby, who, as she is receiving your breastmilk, does not need any remedy against constipation. Even in buying, or having bought for you, such simple everyday medicines like cold-cures it is important to tell the pharmacist you are breastfeeding. Taking aspirin is not safe for any child under 12 and a breastfed baby would get some in your milk.

Visitors

We do have some choice in how we approach the second part of the immediate post-natal period. Some mothers look forward to getting home for some peace, and find that being two plus one is just right. This may not be practical and a mother or mother-in-law, sometimes with their partners, or a sister, or friend, may come to stay or pop round each day. This, in itself, can actually add stress, as well as being a great relief practically. Another person does not know just how you like your toast and where the spaghetti is kept. It is probably best to regard the time as an opportunity to hibernate with the baby.

The ideal helper would be encouraging and knowledgeable about breastfeeding, a cordon bleu cook, have the tact of a diplomat, and love your new family more than anyone else while remaining usefully objective – an almost impossible set of requirements. It is good to have a calm person around, yet you need to know that any worries are not dismissed as trivial. A new grandparent, as well as cooking and shopping, and stopping you from being inundated with too many visitors, especially germy ones, also has to get used to a new place in the family for herself or himself, especially if this is the first grandchild. What you do will be very different from what they did, and their own experiences will come flooding back to them vividly. When they say, 'In our day we used to . . . ' for the twentieth time, it can annoy you: but they may be quite envious of disposable nappies.

Support and advice

This is something you will get a lot of. Some of it may be very useful but needs to be tested to see if it fits your own circumstances, as well as making sense with the facts as you understand them. Support and advice are definitely not the same thing and having someone on your side – whatever happens – is tremendously important.

If family, friends or health professionals comment on nappies or buggies this is not quite so personal as anything they say about how you are feeding the baby. Breastfeeding is something the mother does and she is probably going to get the brunt of any comments made. Twenty-five or so years ago feeding was done very differently indeed, particularly in hospital. All kinds of emotions may come into play when your mother or your partner's other sees you feeding your baby whenever she cries, and doing it for a short or long time, with hours or just half an hour in between. Feeding on one side only at a time, if this is what the baby wants, may seem very strange to her. You may be able to explain all the reasons why you are doing this, rather than limiting feeds to four-hourly intervals, but a previous generation may still feel it is undisciplined, and bad for you and the baby, or simply an indication of something being wrong: 'My mother-in-law told me he was quite simply "starving" and needed to be put on the bottle, something she had done with all three of her sons as they were all "too big" to breastfeed. In my naivety I let her

---

'Sheer stubbornness and a supportive sister-in-law kept me going.'

'So much confusing and conflicting advice!'

'Bottle-feeding would have meant that anyone could feed them. I prefer to get friends to shop or clean for me.'

---

practically force-feed him a bottle of formula milk (I say force-feed as he was only used to the breast and didn't really know what to do with the teat) . . . however – I went to see my health visitor the next day . . . she weighed him and found out he'd been gaining weight quite steadily since birth.'

It can help to get another person talking about what they did in some detail rather than rush to defend your own position – when people are heard carefully they will often explain their own distress at having to pace the floor until the hours were up. You can understand this but still feel very demoralised by the remarks of others. Sometimes you may feel that if only you could convince them that you are right, you will be able to get on with things much better. This is asking a lot. You may just have to get support for what you know is right, from up-to-date profession-als, from your partner, other relatives and friends, and live with the fact that someone you still see often and still love has got stuck on this particular part of being a mother. It may be that in some months, when she sees how well your baby is doing, and how you are not totally drained, she will see for herself what the truth is. Occasionally, this will be a focus for real differences of a deep nature. But, in the end, this is your baby, and you, your partner and those who you trust should come to joint decisions.

Many mothers, even if they have not found breastfeeding easy or happy, can still offer you what you need, if they under-stand what went wrong for them: 'My mother was very sup-portive, even though she herself had "run out of milk" (because of four-hourly feeding regimes).'

Helping does not give people the right to tell you what to do, and nor does their helping mean you must be a parent in the way in which they were. Some direct advice may be right, and some wrong, and many women find what really helps is being listened to carefully while they explore their own ideas and then make up their own minds.

Fathers

Your partner may have all kinds of feelings about breastfeeding and the way it affects you. He may be proud: 'I knew my hus-band enjoyed seeing John and I in our familiar pose, and that he was proud of my efforts.' Or he may be embarrassed, concerned for you if things are getting off to a shaky start, feel excluded in not being able to feed the baby himself, relieved about night feedings and helpless when the baby cries. It can be very hard if your partner is not able to help you in the way you would have liked, for example by saying, 'You were the one who decided to do it . . . ' or by being out all the time, or even by being so upset for you that he finds it hard to allow you to try in case you fail.

If someone is finding it difficult to cope with your breast-feeding even in your own home, you may have to think hard about your approach and it may take time to change things. Your partner can experience a sense of being far less important to you than before as you have fallen in love with a new person, however much he too delights in your new baby. His ability to bath and cuddle the baby, comfort her to sleep when nearness to you makes her think only of milk, may reassure him he is still very much a parent too. One father might make sandwiches ready for your middle of the night feed – it is amazing how hungry you can be at 4am when you have already been up twice since bedtime. Another may find your soreness is only tolerable if he wakes too to talk you through the first moments of the feed.

'I soon found myself banished to the bedroom at feeding time when guests came . . . if I could, I would sit on a dining room chair with my back to my guests so I could join in the conversation . . . as my confidence grew, I certainly did not put up with this sort of nonsense . . . my husband has now changed his attitude and is no longer embarrassed after many heated discussions.'

Remember that he tends to see only the most difficult early period, and then after returning to work, the grizzly evenings, and has not yet seen how any problems calm down and how a more predictable pattern emerges. You may both wonder if you will ever be able to manage to cook and eat and talk to each other as you used to. If you already have one or more children,

What you are offering the family by breastfeeding

- ideal and cheaper food for the baby
- a free arm for stirring, comforting another child, etc
- the possibility of an undisturbed night's sleep for all but mother
- a baby who is less likely to be ill
- instant peace when the baby is hungry, thirsty or miserable
- less smell in nappies and if she is sick

your partner may be busy keeping the toddler happy, and you may feel you have to make an appointment to talk. It is worth making time to speak in peace and to try to find some time for you to spend with the toddler, and for your partner to share with the new baby too, before he returns to work, if that is the plan. Extra complexities arise where there is a second marriage and you and your partner already have children to care for, and other ideas of what mothering and fathering might be like. Some NCT branches do have groups for step-parents to get together and share the joys and challenges of their varying situations. Similarly, if you are bringing up your baby on your own, it may be more important for you to find people in the same situation as yourself as early as you can. In some areas the NCT runs Postnatal Discussion Courses where mothers can share their experiences in facilitated groups.

Getting help from outside the family

The quality of the help available once you are at home will vary just as much as it did in hospital.

'My community midwives were superb and came in most days till Rachel was three weeks old. They never once suggested I give up trying to breastfeed.'

'I spent a very distraught weekend trying to feed my baby myself but she cried incessantly and consequently so did I. A midwife came to visit me (not my own however) and announced "This child is hungry." She stood over me whilst I sterilised a bottle by boiling it and made up a feed. Because my baby slept so soundly as a result, my confidence in my ability to breastfeed was completely eroded.' (This mother continued bottles throughout six months of feeding.)

There can seem a thousand questions to ask and only one visiting midwife to pile them on to – a list may help. After ten days the midwife will usually hand over to the health visitor who will visit less often but be available by phone. She will have an interest in you and your children for several years, and can get to know you quite well, seeing the feeding long-term as a part of your whole mothering. Your own GP may visit you at some point too, and, of course, if you are worried about the baby you can make an appointment to see him or her or ask for a home visit. Surveys have confirmed the impression of many mothers that, sadly, another health professional may bring yet another conflicting piece of advice.* Local groups of community health professionals are increasingly likely to have had further training in breastfeeding, and the Baby Friendly Initiative mentioned earlier gave its first award to a Community Trust in 1999, so there may be a more coherent approach in the future. Meanwhile, where there is a conflict you may find it helpful to talk over what you what to do with a breastfeeding counsellor. With your permission only, it can be helpful for volunteers and professional carers to work together to help you.

The National Childbirth Trust has over 500 qualified and trainee breastfeeding counsellors in Great Britain, available free to *anyone* who wants to get in touch with them. You do not have to be a member of the Trust. Try looking up National Childbirth Trust in the phonebook or writing to the headquarters (see page 192). They do not give medical advice, but they have all fed their own babies, sometimes with problems which they will have now put behind them. They have also done extensive training in how breastfeeding works and ways in which it can go wrong. They can offer information, time, and support for mothers, whatever their concern in relation to breastfeeding, from sore nipples to queries about returning to work. If you both feel the problem is to do with positioning the baby, a visit may seem sensible. If you have been bottle-feeding and decide that you want to change back to breastfeeding, it is often possible to begin again. There are ideas for how to do this in Chapter 13.

'By the time I got home I was crying with pain at each feed. An infection set in causing mastitis and feeding became harder and harder. It was then that we contacted the breastfeeding counsellor. She was my "saving grace". Having spent time with us showing me different positions to hold the baby, I actually felt the baby "drawing" off the milk, for the first time. She was latched on properly at last!'

Breastfeeding counsellors are human too, however: 'no counsellors were available except one who dropped in on her way to her holidays. I am sorry to say all she gave me was a few tips.'

Any conversations with a counsellor are in confidence and do not involve listening to yet more pieces of advice. Instead, counsellors offer information, and try to follow what the mother wants to do, making suggestions to help her. Ideally, breastfeeding counsellors should never say 'you should' or 'you must', but listen to you, give explanations, and offer some strategies for you to choose from, and leave it to you to decide. It would be sad too, if any woman felt she could not contact an NCT breastfeeding counsellor when she is thinking of changing to the bottle. Help is available for ways of doing this without risking feeling too much discomfort.

One of the most helpful things a counsellor can do is to say that she does not know the answer to your query, but refer you on to someone else who does, from the range of expertise available to the Trust. Also, mothers with babies in splints, or with cleft palates, those who have had caesareans or twins and many more may find it useful to ring and be put in touch with someone either locally, or nationally, with a similar experience.

If you do end breastfeeding before you feel ready to do so, you may still feed sad about what happened months or years later, and a breastfeeding counsellor can offer counselling skills to help listen to these feelings too. There is more about ending before you want to in Chapter 13.

The end of the beginning?

Around ten days or a fortnight after the birth can feel like rather a special time. You stop counting the baby's life in days, and usually your helpers begin to disappear, back into their own families, work, or the next mother who needs help. You may begin to feel like a person once more, depending on how things went at the birth, although the midwife can keep calling until 28 days, if necessary.

If the departure of your special helper at this time leaves you alone, either temporarily while your partner is working away from home, or as a single parent or widow, you may now feel particularly unsupported. But there are hundreds of other mothers around and it is to this network which all mothers can now start to look, as an addition to the expertise of the well-informed health professional.

'The only panic I did have was the second night when he kept crying and was very distressed. I tried everything, assuming it was probably the dreaded colic I had heard about. However, eventually I thought as a last resort I'll try and feed him. It turned out he was hungry and I then discovered from talking to my visiting midwife and other mums that this often happens whilst breastfeeding. I spent most evenings thereafter feeding Timothy every half an hour to an hour.'

Myths about breastfeeding

Like many superstitions, you will find that the main nonsenses about breastfeeding often contain numbers. There are already three of them in the good old myth that says 'You must feed on two breasts, for ten minutes each every four hours.' By now you probably know why these arbitrary and unhelpful instructions helped the experts of 50 or 60 years ago to feel that they had done as much as possible to control something which is otherwise in the rather unreliable hands of women and babies. These particular rules are gradually being removed by research, and women's refusal to take a lot of notice. Unfortunately, there is nevertheless a dreadful tendency for rules to creep back constantly into anything to do with infant feeding. For example, once people had heard about it being possible for too much foremilk to be offered by giving two short feeds on both breasts, some hospitals changed their policy to say that all women should feed only on one side at a time.

Some very out of date and misleading information has appeared in publications for mothers in the past and still occasionally slips through. The impression can be given by pictures of expensive food, for example, that you have to eat in a special way to breastfeed, which is not true. You will probably feel hungrier, but extra snacks will be fine. It is a good idea to take with a pinch of salt any set timings suggested in books or magazines. You will sometimes see various claims, about the time it takes for babies to get most of the milk available in each breast, for instance, which suggest that feeds should be time-limited. If a mother has a quick let-down, her milk flows fast and the baby is an eager feeder, the time taken to feed will be shorter than that of another mother and baby pair. But setting a precise timing on a feed can mean that a baby does not get as much increasingly creamy milk as she needs before being put on the other breast or back in her cot. Timings like this are not at all geared to the fact that a newborn baby may feed for half an hour on each breast, while a three-month-old baby may have finished feeding in under ten minutes. In addition, variations in individual feeding patterns throughout a day are enormous, and will depend on appetite. Each baby and mother responds individually. You may find that one baby may get from her mother all she needs in half the time that it takes another mother to transfer the same amount of milk or the same amount of calories to her baby. If feeds are taking a very long time and running into one another for longer than a couple of days, as in a 'growth spurt', you might like to look again at positioning and attaching your baby as effectively as you can, especially if you are sore.

The things people say

'My milk just went overnight.'

It is very unlikely that your grandmother's, aunt's or friend's milk just 'went' overnight. Even when mothers have decided to stop breastfeeding, on the basis of careful thought after a long struggle, they still often find milk remains in their breasts for a long time. Perhaps this mother was trying to feed four-hourly and the baby was sensibly asking for more. Perhaps then she tried to express and nothing came (even though it was there for the baby). Perhaps her breasts felt normally soft after normal fullness at first. So she panicked and bottle-fed – the best she could do with the information she had.

'I only fed four-hourly and no night feeds.'

Complements of formula were normal 20 years ago, helping babies to last four hours. Such timing limited breastfeeding, and both breasts had to be used. Mothers often caved in and accepted bottle-feeding as preferable to sore nipples or pacing the floor with a screaming baby who was not due to feed for an hour and a half. Those who succeeded presumably had babies who wanted to feed ten minutes to a side every four hours – they do occasionally exist – or else they cheated! They may tell you that although they only fed the baby every four hours they did sometimes 'top him up' with a little something in between.

'Your milk must be thin if she needs feeding every two or three hours.'

The milk of a particular mother cannot be 'too thin' – that is, thinner than other mothers' milk – though if you are just offering two short feeds on each breast, it may be quite hard for your baby to get the rich creamy white goodness. Ensure the baby has every opportunity to reach the hindmilk and she may go longer, but two or three hours is OK anyway. It may help to know – and to pass on to others – that in many other cultures babies feed much more often, including during the night, for a long time and that breastfeeding works well without a lot of time rules.

'Your milk will go if you don't rest'

Stress actually raises the level of prolactin (the milk-making hormone) in the body. The prolactin also rises at night, as a part of your normal daily hormone cycle.

Only sudden acute emotions are likely to interrupt breast-feeding, and it is not clear if this is to do with the slowing of let-down of breastmilk or with the baby picking up on distress in the mother. Whatever the cause, the interruption is unlikely to last long. Some milk is available for the baby all the time, even without let-down, and if you let out your distress by crying or talking to someone – even if it is just to the baby to explain what is happening – you will usually find the milk begins to flow again or the baby calms to feed. There is no need to worry about damaging your milk supply or that you are not getting enough rest. Lack of rest can make you feel miserable, but there is no evidence that it does anything to milk supply. If you have been awake a couple of times in the night and have only one baby, you can catch up in the day when she sleeps. If you find it hard to rest during the day even when you are tired, you might find a good time is just after a feed, when you may feel particularly sleepy, like the baby – the effect of hormones on you both. Doing something for yourself such as listening to music, sleeping, eating, jogging, having a long bath, or whatever you feel you need for a while each day probably helps more than twitching dutifully on the settee watching the dust build up. Most people in our society now have some kind of leisure activity, from pottery to karate, and once you are able to get out, there is no reason why a mother has to be totally selfless in her daily life. This can begin with ten minutes uninterrupted reading or gardening with someone else holding the baby. If you are a tidy person who cannot bear any disruption to your normally high standard of house-cleaning, it may help to do the bit where you feed. Decide what your priorities really are, e.g. the sink and lavatories, or the hall and stairs, and just stick to these mainly and let the rest move down the list. If you just cannot bear the place not to be impeccable, then bear in mind that working will not send your milk away, but ignoring the baby, using a dummy a lot and putting off feeds she wants, can mess up your milk supply, so you feel you need complements, or decide that you would be happier with bottle-feeding.

'If I had blocked ducts, mastitis last time, or (much more unusually) an abscess, then I will be more likely to have the same problem again.'
Some women find that the second time they feed their babies they have fewer problems anyway, with experience on their side, but of course you may find problems recurring. It can be useful to find time before you begin feeding again to look carefully at why the breastfeeding went wrong last time, with the help of someone who is interested and may have useful information, like a midwife, health visitor, or breastfeeding counsellor. In this way, you may be able to avoid similar circumstances this time. For example, you may realise that in some way you were not letting one part of your breast be used fully by the baby. Simple ways of clearing a blockage whenever you felt the very beginnings of the problem so as to avoid it getting a real hold may also never have been suggested to you before. You can feel much more in control if you have some strategies for helping yourself.

'If you have fair skin or red hair, you are more likely to get sore nipples.'
This has been disproved. It sounded like a reason for western women's failure in comparison with women from elsewhere, but anyone, of whatever skin colour, can get sore if the baby is not well positioned at the breast. Women and their helpers who had got used to bottle-feeding positions for the baby were treating the nipple like a teat, and so were encouraging sore nipples. This was less likely to happen in places where bottles were not so common.

'My mother, or sister, or friend, couldn't breastfeed, so probably I won't be able to.'
We are not being selectively bred for lactation like dairy cows, and our capacity to breastfeed is very unlikely to be hereditary. It is far more likely that there was a 'good' reason why someone in the past was not able to allow the baby to get the system to work properly. They may have been restricting the time at the breast, or

have been shown incorrectly how to help the baby to feed well. It is likely that when you have read this book or other up-to-date material, and understand how breastfeeding works, that you can make sense for yourself of the person's experience. At a rational level you may then understand that, with good help, the same will not be true for you and your baby, but actually believing this when you have heard or go on hearing about others' difficulties may make it hard for you to trust in breastfeeding.

If you find you are feeling uncertain, despite the baby growing well, this can be because your lack of confidence is still there, and you may find it helpful to talk to someone about this, to put it in perspective. Breastfeeding has been called a 'confidence trick', and it is hard sometimes to find someone who can help you to have trust in your own capacity to make milk.

'Giving your breasts a rest from a feed will store up milk for next time.'

Breastfeeding does not work like this. You cannot 'save' breast-milk inside your body. You will make less overall if you try to make the baby wait long periods between feeds by jiggling her, and especially if you offer alternatives, even like water. In the short-term you feel fuller because you missed a feed, but your body will respond by making less milk, as if the baby needs less – next time you won't be as full (see page 34 for more details about how this works). Milk cannot just 'run out', unless you tell the breasts to make less by not letting the baby, hand or pump remove it. It may help to remember that the breasts are more like a vegetable garden than a freezer. If you keep picking runner beans more keep coming as the plant tries to make seeds for itself, whereas if you take frozen vegetables from the freezer you can run out. Unless you tell your breasts to make less, they will go on making the right amount for your baby.

What is the reason for all these myths about breastfeeding?

It is interesting to think about why there are so very many destructive myths about breastfeeding, although everyone else also tells you what a good thing it is (usually adding 'IF you can do it'). There do not seem to be anywhere near the number of myths about other parts of our biological lives, and those that we hear often sound so silly that we reject them, like burnt toast giving you curly hair, because we realise that they are just a ploy for getting us to do something we do not want to do.

You will find many other examples throughout this book, and in your own lives. They include suggestions about the need to offer extra fluid, the way breastmilk might be frightened away by shocks, and so on. Some of them have grains of truth, which need sieving out from rather a lot of chaff – for example, a baby in hot weather may need extra fluid, but of course it can be breastmilk. Shocks can slow down your ability to allow milk into your baby, but not permanently. Most of them suggest that your breastmilk or your breasts could be in some way inadequate. Time rules also question babies' and mothers' abilities to organise breastfeeding without lots of interference, and show a basic suspicion of the way in which breastfeeding works. They all need questioning in the light of your own real experience as well as research.

It seems a great pity that there needs to be so much explanation about how breastfeeding works, whereas we just expect our digestive system to turn our food into energy without understanding about the chemical and physiological workings of our insides on what we eat. But there is no readily available alternative for 'real' food which is acceptable to everyone, as there is for breastmilk – we have not quite got to the stage of eating a few pills to keep ourselves going like in science fiction.

Many people drive quite happily without knowing how an engine works and do not mind taking it all on trust – until the car breaks down. We often have a trust in the workings of manmade objects which we do not feel for women's 'products', so it is worth trying to understand a little about how the process happens. Breastfeeding has been a tried and tested method of feeding throughout history – quite a lot of 'Research and Development' – and where things do go wrong, this is usually not because of built-in design defects in the system or in us as individuals, but because there are one or more 'spanners in the works', often based on such myths as those above, which you may need help to find and remove.

CHAPTER SEVEN

Day to day breastfeeding

*'I also remember when Louise was three or four
weeks old, listening to a friend with a baby about six
weeks old, who told me that at last she was feeling
settled with the feeding. I found it very reassuring
that she too had found it quite hard for the first few
weeks, but that by about six weeks, things had
changed. It took us about that long to feel
that we'd got it right.'*

Once you and the baby are left to get on with life you will become
fully aware of what a big change in lifestyle you are having to
adjust to without any training to help you. Feeling at home with
feeding takes each mother and baby a different length of time.

At first, you may be lonely once your partner or mother has
gone, and yet too busy too feel bored. Each day can seem very
long without the time being divided up as it was perhaps in hospital or in your work. This is even more obvious if you have no
one coming home each day, because they are working at home,
out of work, or you are a single parent. You may feel you have
very little to show for the day's effort, and what is done will have
to be done again tomorrow. No wonder a new mother can seriously wonder, despite the love she feels for her baby, if she is
somehow 'trapped'. You may feel the need to recreate a structure
by listing tasks and ticking them off, or even, as one mother did,
setting a timer to go off regularly so she at least felt aware of the
passage of time.

You may very much miss the company of other adults, particularly if you are not as able to get out as you would like perhaps because you are still recovering from a caesarean, or you are a wheelchair user. It may be a help to use the telephone, if you have one, to get in touch with other mothers in similar situations, to talk over the birth, and to build up a network of people to share experiences with.

This may also be a good time to reassess your priorities in looking after the house; cooking, washing and all the other jobs which have to be done. It is hard to believe that feeding, bathing, and changing one very small person could possibly take so long. It may help to write down all you do in a day. 'I had assumed with an average gap of four hours between feeds, I'd have at least three hours in which to do other things, but this was not true at all.' If your standards have always been high, it may be difficult to have to interrupt a task and make time to feed the baby. Interruptions are the norm from now on – later it will be potties and the endless questions of a child who is learning to speak. It is your home and you are the one who probably spends most time in it now, so you can rethink any routines you set out with. A baby does not need a bath every day, and it need not happen in a morning. People have been known to bath their babies at midnight as long as the room is warm enough, knowing that after a bath she would feed well and then sleep.

Everything about having had a baby makes you feel distinctly different, and especially breastfeeding. Most of what you do with your baby now is feed her and so this comes to be a tremendous focus for your attention. If it is going well, there can be great delight in the drunken looking baby who falls of your breast after softly gulping a good feed: if not, times at the breast can become a struggle, repeated over and over again, perhaps half a dozen times while you are on your own, and then – often at its worst – when your partner comes home.

Patterns in the baby's day

While the baby is very young, you may not be meeting many other mothers, but they would almost all be saying that the evenings are the worst time of the day. Everyone is tired, and now the baby wants to feed continuously without a proper sleep, perhaps from 7 till 10, or 5 till 8 – the permutations are endless – and the main aim seems to be to prevent you from making or eating a main meal together in peace. One strategy is to try to cook in the morning if you get a chance, putting on a slow casserole and not relying on being able to make a meal in half an hour like you did when you got in from work. Chop and chips may have left the menu for a while. If you remember how active your baby probably was while still in your womb when you sat down at the end of the day, you may find that this stage is easier to understand.

Different writers offer different explanations for the grizzly behaviour so common in babies of this age at this time of day. Some say it is nervous excitability, while others believe it is an attempt to fill their tummies repeatedly with lots of milk, so as to try, however inadequately for now, to sleep longer at night, it may give you some hope, while you just put your feet up, watch television, and feed and hold the baby. She perhaps cannot eat very well because she is fidgety and tired, like you in a motorway cafe at 1am, needing to eat to drive on, but wanting really to sleep.

Knowing roughly what to expect can help, although all babies are very different. Usually you can rely on the baby to want at least six or seven feeds during a day, and to wake quite early in the morning, after one or two feeds in the night. In all this, the pattern of the baby's feeding and sleeping is as yet often scarcely visible. One day may be suddenly warmer and she wants short, frequent feeds of foremilk, crying after a few moments on one breast. This does not mean there is no milk left. If you offer the other side she will take it and you may find she wants the same again in another hour and a half. Or it will suddenly turn cold, and after a walk to the shops, the baby is so hungry that she feeds and feeds – both sides and then wants more. Don't panic. There *is* more, already being made in the first side while she feeds on the second. So put her back on the first side, then the second and keep going if necessary. She may want seconds of all the courses available today. Another day, she is filled easily from milk she has called up in you – milk you may have felt suddenly to be there in a big way after two hard days of extra feeds. Like ours, her appetite varies with the work she is doing – all that smiling, waving, just being, makes her extra hungry sometimes in one of the growth spurts you can expect, at around three or six weeks, or any time the baby is ready to move on.

You may never know for certain, or even at all, what has caused the changes in the feeding pattern of a baby. If it worries you, talk to someone, but do be careful of advice which too quickly leaps to the bottle as a solution. Of course, a bottle of formula will fill up a hungry baby who is working hard to increase your milk supply over two days or so and stop her from trying to improve things. It will also be less good at satisfying the thirst of the baby who is hot – water would be better for that. But you have perfectly good foremilk full of vitamins and energy-producing sugars for a thirst-quenching drink for a miserable baby, so it simply is not necessary to give bottles of boiled water.

Weighing

Finding out for sure that the baby is growing steadily can be a great reassurance that she is well, and you are getting the hang of feeding together. You are looking for an overall pattern, with possible dips and flat parts to the graph when the baby is a little off-colour, or in hot weather, and so on. You will need to wait for a few visits to the clinic before you can see the true pattern of your baby's growth again, as she will be weighed on yet another set of scales.

'His weight gain was constantly enormous and due to certain close family pressure, I was a regular clinic attender to "prove" that his apparent appetite did not indicate that my milk supply was inadequate.'

Babies can have quite large motions and also lose a lot of weight in urine just before weighing, or seem to jump up in weight after a big feed, so you are looking at averages, not just what each difference is from day to day, or even week to week. A baby can seem to be staying quite still on the chart and then make a big gain. On the whole, breastfed babies do seem to put weight on in a less regular way than bottle-fed ones – with more at first, sometimes up to a pound a week, dropping to less than the average bottle-fed baby at around four months. It is a shame that the charts which are still being used to judge the gain of the babies in this country were actually drawn up at a time when most babies were being bottle-fed and so had a different sort of curve on their graphs. There is some evidence that, whether bottle-fed or breastfed, babies who are considered to be growing considerably under the average amount may be smaller as children without suffering any measurable intellectual or educational damage.* Not all breastfed babies gain weight so quickly at first – some gain around 3–4 oz a week steadily. A second baby may not grow at the same rate as her big brother or sister, so making comparisons is not helpful.

Motions may now begin to be more infrequent, and not even happen daily. If the baby does wait several days she may sometimes feed rather irritably before the great moment arrives. Urine still needs to give plenty of wet nappies, and it should be clear.

Being sick

If the baby brings up a little bit of curdled milk on top of wind this is mainly a nuisance for carpets and cardigans. If it looks as though 'the whole feed' has come back, all you can do is wait to see if the baby gets hungry soon, but it usually looks a lot more than it is and there will be milk being made already so there is no need to offer bottled milk. If she is very sick, especially with vomits which whoosh across the room for some distance, you will want to see your health visitor or doctor for reassurance, explanations or treatment (see Chapter 9).

Distress

One minute's crying in a baby, especially if nothing you try makes any difference, can feel like an hour, and an hour like a week. If you are alone at home you can wait for the crying to start as if your ears are out on long sensitive feelers. This is perhaps why our grandmothers put the baby down the garden. Now it is more likely that the baby is near at hand and every squirm and snuffle sounds loud and worrying.

Sometimes babies get into a cycle of taking very short frequent feeds which quench their thirst and give them enough energy from the sugar in the milk to keep going. These drinks do not fill them up as longer feeds that reach the hindmilk might do. There are good times to give lots of little feeds. A regular three- to four-hour gap between all feeds is not something many small babies have – any more than adults do! Most little babies take small frequent feeds all evening, and that is normal. Your baby may be hot because of a sudden change in the weather or because she is just a bit off colour. A baby who is going through a growth spurt will feed practically non-stop for a day or so too.

However, lots of little feeds may lead to tummy ache, and another feed to calm the baby just makes it all worse. If feeding goes on endlessly – especially if it is in the night as well – it may be worth having a couple of days where you try other ways of comforting the baby – rocking, walking, hoovering and so on – so that she gets the experience of hunger followed by a really good meal to see if she prefers this way of eating. This is not the same as letting your breasts fill up 'properly' (you may well give more food by little feeds); it is just to see if this pattern helps you and the baby to be less miserable. If the penny doesn't drop with her you could just continue to 'go with the flow' for a while – it can be much harder to rock and walk than just to sit down and feed and wait for the baby to sort it all out.

Although the sensible thing is to try feeding first you may be finding this is not always now the answer. Talking, cuddling, stroking and other interactions begin to be important too. There is so little a baby of this age can do for herself to keep herself cheerful, you can feel as if you have very little peace.

Continuing to look after yourself

Looking after yourself is necessary because you matter, not just to the family. Recovering from childbirth needs good nutrition. If for some reason you were unable to keep yourself up to your normal weight, breastfeeding would continue, but the baby would take more and more, usually shorter, feeds.

The trouble with missing meals or having a poor diet yourself is that you begin to feel tired, and low in energy, and may be more prone to picking up illnesses. Most mothers find that while they are breastfeeding, they are hungrier and yet can still lose weight or maintain it. It is so easy to miss breakfast, forget to stop in the middle of washing to have a coffee break, snatch a late and skimpy lunch. Then you can be so busy all afternoon that you have no time to make yourself something nourishing before you launch into cooking a large meal for the family or you and your partner. Even then you don't get a chance to eat this in peace because babies are often awake and miserable around the time that most people eat.

Spreading out your intake of food through the day, as perhaps you felt you needed to do when you were first pregnant to stop yourself feeling too sick, and at the end of pregnancy when there was not room for a big meal, can be a very useful habit to continue while you breastfeed. You do need some extra calories, but the process of making milk is very efficient and happens with a lot less extra energy being used than was previously thought.

You may well feel hungry, but if you are finding that caring for the baby is making you worried, you may miss the signals before your stomach is churned up and you cannot distinguish between the hole of hunger and the knots of anxiety. Talk to someone about your feelings – your health visitor, doctor or breastfeeding counsellor may be able to help there. Food to make milk does not have to be special, or even cooked, so sandwiches are fine. Whatever you eat will turn into breastmilk, still following the recipe which, as always, is just right for your baby.

Dieting

People often tell you that when you breastfeed you get your figure back. However, many mothers feel they have borrowed someone else's figure while they are feeding their babies! Breastfeeding does mean that your womb will get back to its normal size more quickly after the baby is born, although your breasts will be bigger, especially in the first few weeks of the baby's life. Breastfeeding mothers usually have bigger appetites and need to eat some extra calories. This usually happens just by you responding to feeling more hungry and thirsty. These extra calories are less than the energy value of the milk the baby takes, as breastfeeding women are efficient at making adult food into

Some reminders about you and your food

- If you find yourself becoming constipated, you may need to drink more but usually you can rely on your own thirst.
- Drinking milk itself is not a necessity – no other mammal does it. You need calcium, but milk products like yoghurt and cheese can supply that and baked beans, bread, nuts and tinned fish with bones in it like sardines contain it too.
- Your diet needs to be good to look after a baby, however you are feeding her, with fresh fruit, vegetables and so on, but there is no need to eat a lot of extra protein.
- It may help to eat often – don't try to last out for long periods while you are offering her lots of little feeds. It can make you feel 'drained'. Even at night, if you are doing a couple of feeds, you may feel hungry.

milk for babies. Some women find they can eat very well and still lose weight gained during pregnancy as they breastfeed while others do not lose weight until they finish breastfeeding. You may feel you need to diet, and if you do this by avoiding the foods that we all know are not good for us, it will not affect your milk supply. You have to be really malnourished before the quantity of milk is affected. Your baby will take care of the balance in the meal she gets from you, so the quality of your feeds will stay the same; that is, they will go on being just what the baby needs at that particular time, whether she is more or less active and growing steadily or fast. However, you can feel low if you are giving milk several times a day without snacks. Limiting your intake of food can make you feel that breastfeeding is draining, which is a shame. There is also some research to suggest that if you diet hard you begin to mobilise your own fat stores to make some parts of the milk. There is then the possibility that any contaminants that may be stored in your fat, such as dioxins, can more easily transfer to the milk. If you feel you must diet you can get expert help from a dietician via your GP, and you may like to talk over the issue with a breastfeeding counsellor.

Will it upset the baby?

There are all kinds of myths about what you should and should not eat while you are breastfeeding. If you feel something is upsetting the baby, you could try removing it from your diet for a week, to see if it makes any difference. Do talk this over with a health professional if it is a big and important item such as cow's milk as this needs a lot of thinking about. A breastfeeding counsellor can supply a cow's milk free diet sheet.

Relaxation

You may be remembering to do some postnatal exercises now, and perhaps it is useful to remind yourself of the value of relaxation not just during feeding but also when you are chopping onions and find your shoulders are up around your ears. It is OK if you are deliberately using the onions to remove aggression or tension, but the extra work is tiring as a habit.

Milk supply

The main concern which mothers still have at this time in feeding, when they have hopefully sorted out any sore nipple problems (if not, see page 54), is the one which people constantly remind you of – 'Have you enough milk?' The usual ways of knowing still work – the way the baby is, that what goes in must come out, and that a steady average weight gain of anything from 3 oz upwards a week is fine.

People may tell you that the baby is feeding all the time because you are now up and about and the activity is reducing your milk supply. However, women who are still in hospital and in bed for a good deal because of infections and so on notice just the same sorts of increasing demands, and as you know, it is not doing things which somehow frightens away milk, but not feeding long enough or effectively enough. Here are some of the things which may make you feel that you haven't enough milk and some ideas about them.

- fist sucking – this is just something that babies do as there is not a lot else they can do to amuse themselves. It means nothing about your milk supply.
- softer breasts – these are normal. If you are not producing surplus milk, you are responding more accurately to what she wants. Leaking often stops after a few weeks as you and the baby match demand and supply more accurately.
- the baby is hungry all the time, or does not settle – she may be having a growth spurt, but if it is all the time, check the position again.
- she will take a bottle – lots of babies will, but it doesn't mean they were actually needing it.
- she is not growing well – get help with improving your milk supply and check that all is well with the baby herself. If you lost a lot of blood around the time of the birth, your midwife or doctor may offer extra iron, as there is some evidence that anaemia can make it harder at first to produce the milk your baby needs. Very occasionally a woman who has fragments of placenta in her womb can find making a full milk supply difficult until these fragments leave her body, as her hormones are telling her she is still pregnant. Both these conditions can be treated.

'I think it's true that it takes several weeks to really establish feeding. It was amazing that for quite a few weeks I still wasn't sure if I would have enough milk to feed him when he was hungry again. My fears were not borne out by my community midwife who was extremely supportive and brought her students to see me because she thought I was a shining example of good breastfeeding. Being on my own, this extra care from her was most welcome.'

Other things to offer?

Bottles

It is often suggested that a bottle is the 'answer' to any problem about milk supply, especially the one of the tea-time constant feeding. It is easy for babies to become reliant on the instant fix of the bottle, as the milk flows instantly and consistently. Your milk supply is more interestingly varied and the baby must stimulate it by her own efforts. Some babies adapt well to using both methods, for example taking expressed breastmilk from a childminder later. Sometime during this period mothers who are going back to work, or whose partners wish to be involved in feeding, may decide to begin to introduce a regular infrequent bottle, either of expressed breastmilk or water, to try to ensure it is not refused later.

If a bottle is suggested by a health professional, and you wish to continue breastfeeding, do ask for help with increasing your milk supply as well as, or instead of, using formula.

Other liquids

Other people may feel that it is difficult to believe that breastmilk contains all a baby needs. Few would bring round thick broths for four-week-old babies as they did at one time, but you will have various additions suggested. The Department of Health recommends that breastfed babies are given vitamin drops from the age of six months. As this recommendation is based on the need for *some* babies, for example those born prematurely, to get vitamins at this time, Health Trusts will have different ideas about interpreting the guidelines. Some health visitors do not suggest vitamin drops for the baby as long as he or she is taking formula or breastmik as a main source of food. One government report argues that it is important that the mother herself is eating a good diet and recommends that all breastfeeding mothers take supplements, as breastmilk contains all the vitamins that babies need. You could discuss this with your health visitor or a dietician if you are worried about your own diet for any reason.

Dummies

Dummies can obviously be a great boon to a hard-pressed mother. However, many breastfed babies will not accept one with any enthusiasm. They can confuse the baby about sucking and suckling, as bottle teats do. They also may satisfy sucking needs that would be better used stimulating your milk supply. Some research has shown a connection between the use of dummies for more than two hours a day and breastfeeding problems. It may be that the dummies led to the problems or it may be that the problems made the baby miserable and so parents used a dummy, but it is worth thinking hard about whether to give your baby a dummy.

Helping yourself

Housework and feeding can make motherhood feel as if it is something you have to do all by yourself. Going out and talking to other mothers may seem both a practical impossibility and a self-indulgence, but mothers who have experienced early weeks with babies generally find that spending time together is of tremendous benefit. Even if other mothers do seem to be on top of things, you will find that conversations soon reveal that they too can be still in their dressing gowns at 3pm and find evenings difficult.

Asking for help

It may be that when you have looked at all you have to do in a day, it is just not possible without some help from others. Mostly this will be a partner. He may have quickly grown used to your maternity leave and have forgotten a time when you both worked and both shared housework. It is important to be able to negotiate about tasks without feeling that you are having to ask for help in a plaintive way, or to wait until you are so desperate for someone to notice that you are struggling, that you are forced to ask with a tremendous burst of annoyance. It can be harder for a partner to realise the changes in your lives. His going off to play rugby or sitting down after tea to watch the news while you, who made the meal, wash up as well, may just be habits. The baby may love a harder shoulder, a deeper voice, and a different height of the wall to look at, but you may feel guilty that as soon as your partner walks in, tired too, he is handed a baby to hold.

As you settle into a week to week pattern of life, it is often hard even to find time to reassess your own priorities, you are usually so busy doing them. It can be difficult to talk about these things because the baby is always taking the attention from both of you as well. But without discussion it is hard to decide on what you both feel are the important tasks and who is going to be responsible for getting particular jobs done. Soaking dishes saves a lot of time but does it upset either of you? How important is it to have a meal at a set time or a cooked pudding rather than yoghurt and fruit? If it is a matter of feeling that you would let yourself down in some way, it could be worth thinking about who exactly you are trying to live up to.

Meeting both your needs

You may be making all kinds of assumptions about how the other person feels if the bed is not made. It can be that any concerns about housework, or meals, are actually about your partner feeling that he has unmet needs. Where previously you may have both unloaded your day to each other, you may be so tired, and short of adult company that for the moment, your needs are much greater.

As the first few weeks draw to a close and the baby's age begins to be counted in months the question of resuming a full sexual relationship can cause some difficulty. Research points to all kinds of conflicting findings here. Although women are supposed to find breastfeeding sometimes arousing in itself and it has been claimed that they wish to return to intercourse more quickly, many women are still very tired, and sore, after the birth. They and their partners may find that breasts do seem to be for babies at this point too. They can feel heavy and tender, with leakage likely unless the baby is fed just before lovemaking – itself likely to be interrupted. Different positions for making love, like the 'spoons' position which avoids squashing the woman's breasts may help.

Your needs to recover from broken nights can clash with your partner's needs. There is a range of responses with no right or wrong, simply ones which you are both happy with, and ones in which both or one of you is not happy. You can only know about what you are both feeling by sharing what you think rather than just imagining what the other person may be feeling and avoiding the issue. Just finding time and a place to do this without falling asleep can be really hard with a baby who wakes up at night.

If you both go on being unhappy, talk to someone, perhaps a breastfeeding counsellor may be able to help, and the GP or health visitor can have suggestions. An appointment for family planning advice may also provide a good opportunity for useful discussion about this whole area. It is worth remembering that Relate offers counselling in all relationship difficulties.

Toddlers

Toddlers still need a lot of attention at fairly short notice, and it is hard to breastfeed while pulling up trainer pants. You may remember feeding him and feel he has had his turn and should allow the baby to have your attention first, but realise it is hard for him to wait too. It is easy to fall into the habit of promising time and attention 'soon', and best perhaps to do things with a toddler before trying to do jobs. Involving him does make it less straightforward but can mean it gets done. Feeding cross-legged on the floor, if this is comfortable, can be very good for playing at cars or jigsaws with older children, and it may help to have everything to hand – potty, sultanas in little boxes, fruit juice, a special box of toys, and so on, for the next feed. A video recorder to timeshift suitable programmes is invaluable. Not all babies appreciate mothers who read to toddlers during feeds but it is worth a try.

If your toddler is needing attention, he may find the best way to get it is to be particularly noisy, boisterous, or even violent, during breastfeeds. Some babies quickly learn that the night is the best time to feed in an undistracted way after a while, and extend the quiet feeds – after the toddler is in bed or in the early morning – while cutting down day time feeds to a minimum.

While some babies will feed steadfastly through toys being driven over them, some may become 'fussy' at these feeds, or later pull off and look around at the excitement. Practically, it is not always possible to persuade a toddler to be read to quietly, go to playgroup, or be cared for by a kind neighbour, while getting over the difficult hurdle of bringing in a 'little stranger' who is not part of your first child's plan at all. It may help to have the radio on playing music so that the sudden bangs and shrieks make less sudden impact on the baby.

Even toddlers may have totally forgotten their own feeding experience, so may ask 'why is that baby eating you?' or may want to have a go. If he was bottle-fed you may feel sad that this baby is having something your first child missed out on. If you want to talk about feeding there are some books which will help a toddler see the different ways of feeding and may help him to settle in with a new baby. Some are listed on page 198.

Older children

A lot is often expected of older children, not just by getting them involved in helping, but by expecting them not to mind as much about the new arrival. Of course, they too may feel pushed out but be more subtle in their ways of showing it, and need reassurance that they are still loved for their own sake and not just because they get the nappy cream from upstairs. You may need to spend a lot of time offering other forms of closeness to older children, perhaps reading, bathing together or special cuddles without the baby.

Friends

Unless there was a lot of good timing, it is unlikely that your friends will also be having babies at exactly the right time to fit with yours and so you will be faced with making new relationships as well. What will all the other mothers think of you? Maybe they all seem very at ease with their babies, even if they are only a few weeks older. There is a huge gap between a tiny floppy bundle of two weeks old and a ten-week-old who sits in his mother's arms or a babychair.

Help continued

Anyone may offer blanket reassurance which dismisses your problem: this is never a lot of help. It is less than helpful to suggest to a mother who has a baby who cries all the time – on the breast and between feeds – that the problem will settle down and that breastfeeding is the solution to everything. The baby may be ill, or not feeding in a good position. Try to find someone who knows enough to offer positive suggestions.

Tasks involving the baby is what most helpers want – you can offer bathing or topping and tailing or even nappy changing to the most devoted and trustworthy perhaps. With most offers, it can be hard to say 'What I really need is someone to clean the bathroom.' Shopping with the baby so that you can rest or do something you want – like listen to music or polish the brass – may be really helpful, or the offer of casseroles and ironing which buy you time with the baby and the family. It might help to have a list, in your head or on paper, of tasks you don't ever seem to get round to, in case someone does offer some help.

Health professionals

Midwives hand over to health visitors usually at ten days, although they may visit until 28 days. Health visitors will take responsibility for the 'well baby' parts of your baby's health care, from advice on feeding, vitamin drops and so on, to immunisation and sight and hearing checks until she begins school. You may have her phone number so that you can catch her before she does visits if you are worried about feeding. She will invite you to attend the well baby clinic where you can have the baby weighed, and see a health visitor and possibly a clinic doctor if you wish. It is worth remembering that not all people operating baby scales are qualified health visitors, but may be volunteers. They may encourage you if the baby has gained well, but easily sow the seeds of doubt for a mother whose baby has not put on a lot of weight. If you are worried about any comment, or the actual weight gain or loss, do talk to the health visitor. You may want to ask for help with continuing breastfeeding and perhaps asking for ways of increasing your milk supply, as well as considering seriously any suggestions made about bottles.

'I remember the community midwife saying how well she thought I was coping with the feeding every time she called. Although I did not realise it I started to believe it and felt more confident.'

Where you feel there is more than a minor health problem you, or she, can ask to see your own General Practioner. Do remind your doctor, or dentist, if you are prescribed medicines, that you are still breastfeeding. You can always ring any pharmacist about the compatibility of medicines and breastfeeding too.

Back to normal?

When you have had your postnatal checkup at around 6 weeks after the baby's birth, you may begin to put pressure on yourself, or to feel it coming from elsewhere, to be totally back to your old self. In fact you will never be your *old* self – you are now a mother – rather, a *new* self with new priorities. By now, many women you know will have stopped breastfeeding for various reasons, and you may be beginning a longer breastfeeding journey, feeling a little unsure of the unmarked roads, but ready for a few outings.

For many mothers the next hurdle is returning to work, dealt with in more detail in Chapter 11. If this is happening in such a way that you feel the baby needs to get used to a bottle, then once you feel secure about breastfeeding, your own expressed breastmilk can be given in a bottle (see page 153). Leaving this until much later may make it harder for your baby to learn this new trick, while earlier may disrupt her breastfeeding skills. Whether you are returning to work or simply deciding you must make a dash to the shops, these first steps towards being apart from your baby may be a part of your life from now on.

Chapter Eight

The breastfeeding journey

---

*'I think the nicest time of all is the late night feed
when she's still sleepy and without opening her eyes she
snuffles around trying to find the nipple.'*

The need to learn quickly for the first few weeks of breastfeeding
can make it feel like a big new responsibility. Just as you cannot
risk talking too much or turning your head around when you are
driving a car, you have to keep your eyes – and ears – on standby
all the time for the baby. Once breastfeeding begins to feel a
normal part of daily life, it can clearly become a less demanding
route to have chosen. The stage at which you both feel really
comfortable with breastfeeding will vary from one mother and
baby to another, depending on the nature and number of any
crises and problems you meet.

If for some reason caring for the baby has been an uphill
struggle, you can find the relentless demand for you focuses on
feeding, the one task you cannot delegate. It is the one job you
must sit or lie down to do, however, and it may help to try to
work out whether there are other things which are making you
fed up and tired.

Being with other breastfeeding mothers can be a great help.
You may find them through the clinic, your antenatal class, or
the NCT postnatal support system – anyone can go to any coffee
mornings organised by them. Those at the same stage are able to
share similar feelings, those just behind you can make you feel
really proficient, and those ahead can teach you a lot. You may

notice details like how they do not bother to remember which side to give first but just feel each breast. If neither feels heavier it doesn't matter anyway. Many mothers actually feed their babies far more on one breast than the other if it feels more comfortable for both them and the baby. It is quite possible, as with twins or after some surgery, to feed a baby using just one breast.

---

*'I love watching others doing it.
(Doesn't it sound nice?)'*

Changes

Now that the baby is able to support herself and turn her own head to reach for the breast, you can experiment with different feeding positions. It may be worth trying positions you tested out earlier and did not find comfortable, in case a couple of months' growth and improvement in the baby's muscle tone, as well as your own increased skills, have made any difference. Feeding a baby lying down with large engorged breasts may have felt difficult. Now you may find it a good way to rest.

For some mothers, watching a baby develop solely on their breastmilk is very rewarding. They remember all kinds of different things about breastfeeding.

There are times now when you feel that you have been breastfeeding all your life, and that as it is so easy you are glad you don't have to sterilise or prepare bottles. You are free to pick up the baby and a nappy bag and head for a day out, or a morning with friends. It is like coasting down a long hill to the seaside on a sunny day.

You may find the baby is becoming more adaptable. Demand feeding can work both ways. If you have always responded to your baby right away when she is hungry, she will trust you to come soon if you tell her you are on the way from the ironing board. If going to playgroup to meet an older child, you may need to wake the baby to give her a little drink before you set out, so that she will not be desperate as you walk along. It is worth thinking about where you can feed in such necessary excursions. A teacher or headmistress may be able to find you somewhere quiet after school if your baby is going through a phase where she is easily distracted or if you want privacy for yourself. It is worth asking before you are put in the position of dashing home with a distressed baby or standing in the street uncomfortably feeding. If there are shops or a library nearby, there may be somewhere you can feed the baby. Just knowing that there is somewhere to go if necessary will relieve one anxiety. A friend may live between your home and the school – see how she feels about you dropping in if you need to.

Feeding patterns

As the baby grows and her technique becomes increasingly efficient and your let-down happens more readily, feeds take less time. Some mothers cannot believe that their child can possibly be getting enough with perhaps a five-minute suck. Again this is the time to be reminded that wet nappies and satisfactory weight gains are a good indication of what is going in, provided there is no other fluid being given. You may, despite the amount of milk being produced, feel less aware of both fullness and let-down if you had them earlier. It is as if the engine is now running smoothly, ticking over most of the time very quietly, and ready to move off whenever it is needed.

By about three months, some kind of predictable pattern may be emerging in the baby's sleeping and feeding. She may have an early morning feed, which seems copious and filling, yet want another one quite soon. Foremilk is plentiful in the morning, and provides the equivalent of tea in bed, or orange juice before breakfast. Either before or after elevenses you may be able to count on a 'long' sleep – depending on what your baby's ideas about sleep are, this may be 20 minutes, or three hours, or

---

'Imperceptibly everything changed. Feeds grew shorter, my breasts stopped leaking . . . he started sleeping through the night and I did not feel as if I was constantly feeding him any more. From three to six months everything was perfect, and I wouldn't have missed it for the world.'

---

more. Some babies do a similar thing after lunch – a 'siesta' when you might usefully join in if you have no other children. After that, most babies are snacking and (briefly) dozing, being talked to, or grizzling over and beyond the traditional northern tea times and southern supper times. This is only one possible pattern – your baby may do something quite different.

Having perhaps gained large amounts at first, the baby's weight gain may then slow down at around three months. She will begin to use feeding as an opportunity for a kind of conversation and play rather than just for food and drink, just as we might like to eat in the company of others: 'he plays with the "bosoms" with the same inquisitiveness he explores the rest of the world.'

Feeds in the night

It is not unusual for a baby still to be feeding in the night, and all babies start to 'sleep through' at different times. We all wake up in the night, check that everything is OK, turn over and forget all about it – unless something is wrong, whether that is a pain, thirst or anything else. Some babies do this every two hours or so and call for their mother to help them settle with a short sleep-inducing feed. This is a difficult pattern to break in the night, and it can be helpful to let your baby learn about relaxing into sleep for herself in the day by gradually making sure she is not always dropping off at the breast, but is put down while awake if drowsy. Health visitors can be helpful about this.

Keeping babies happy

Your baby may still, of course, have periods when she cries miserably and needs comforting, but you will now be aware that food is not always the answer. A bored baby needs a lot of talking and entertaining from you or her father.

Feeding outside the home

Your own journeys are much more likely now. Having a friend call for you to take you to a coffee morning of strangers can seem stretching enough at first. You may be the kind of person who has never been to such an event in her life, and wonder what you are doing there, and what everyone else will be like, and think of you. Being up and dressed and organised for a set time may be quite a hurdle. At least this is an event arranged with small children in mind, but other outings bring you up against the real, and very adult-centred world.

---

*'He was fed everywhere – in restaurants, parks,
in the car, on a ferry and a bus, at home and abroad,
and I never heard and adverse comment or had
a disapproving look.'*

Whether it is the first time with the baby to the local swimming baths or the first time without the baby to the decent shops, friends who have been there or are sharing the road with you can be a tremendous help in defusing panic and in reminding you what you might need. Of course, the great benefit of breastfeeding is that the main picnic ingredient is always ready. But it can be a problem deciding where to offer it, and how you will feel. You can solve the problem to some extent by trying to feed discreetly: 'Baggy T-shirts, sweatshirts and jumpers all make it easy to feed without exposing your breasts to all and sundry' or '. . . David refused to be pacified with bread. To soothe his screams I plugged him on, and studied the soup shelves with great concentration for 10 minutes.'

Having someone else with you may help to ease any embarrassment you might feel about your first public feeding experience. The other person can shield you physically from stares perhaps, or act as an extra spokesperson if necessary. You may find places with symbols showing that a mother may feed and change her baby here – often this is a bottle, although some symbols are more open-minded.

You may find that some large stores will quite happily allow you to use a changing room, except at busy times like Saturdays and during sales. Others may have special baby and mother rooms. But you may find it hard to find a welcoming place. Going out, aware that you may need to breastfeed your baby in a public place, can be very worrying for some mothers.

Occasions when women are asked to stop feeding seem to be quite rare but they do make a big impression, and can make others feel rather cautious. 'I did not have the confidence or courage to breastfeed Mark in any public place given society's attitude.'

These problems are not connected with the feeding, but with the reactions of other people. Your own feelings may be quite calm, defensive of your baby and your right to feed, or apprehensive, but what will you say if another customer objects, or an assistant asks you to stop doing it, to go away, or offers you the staff toilet to feed in? It is worth considering these questions before you set out if you are worried.

Mothers have tried these responses:

- explaining – 'My baby will be a lot more noisy crying than feeding, so I am feeding her.'
- repeating calmly to each objection 'My baby needs feeding now.'
- asking 'presumably you would be happy if I were bottle-feeding, so why are you unhappy that I am breastfeeding?' If the reply is that someone may be able to see your breasts you will probably be able to point out that this is not so. Certainly, the nipple is covered by the baby and if you are wearing something fairly loose and separate you can just lift it up to feed. The often recommended shawl or large headscarf is worth considering too, although it is up to you how much you feel you need to vanish.

If you are told to feed in the toilet you may like to explain that you do not consider this a good place to feed a baby. It is not hygienic. No adult would be expected to eat there.

'Articles I have read discourage women from breastfeeding in public by suggesting that it is an activity which shouldn't really be done in a public place but which should be confined to a mother's room, the loo, or the changing cubicles of a shop.'

One keen theatre-goer mother solved her problem by getting her family a box at the theatre.

Separation

Going out without your baby for a while can also be a challenge. There is the question of your own comfort, of course, and it is certainly wise to take extra breast pads, and be prepared to express milk if you feel you will be away for longer than a usual interval between feeds. Without the baby, you may feel a strange mixture of relief and concern, after all the time you spent together, almost as if you have left something behind as important as your handbag. It may seem incredible to you that sometimes mothers later forget which shop they have left the pram outside.

Babysitters

People urge you to go out as a couple and yet it may well be that the only person you know who can calm your baby apart from yourself, is your partner. If he is willing to be the very first babysitter, you could leave some expressed breastmilk and a little spoon and cup. Do not be surprised if this is not quite as good as the real thing and you find on your return a rather wakeful baby. He could practise offering slow sips with you out of the room to allow the baby time to suck the milk off the spoon or out of the cup. A baby who is inundated with milk may be very upset. Similarly, a bottle is best offered by someone else at first.

When you decide that the time has come to set out as a pair, without a baby for a change, and you are going out to something with a timed start, don't be surprised if the baby seems to sense that you are in a hurry to leave and takes extra time over the feed before you go. It can help to leave yourself lots of time for this feed. Babysitters obviously need to know just where you are in case the baby is inconsolable.

More challenging journeys

Holidays bring mothers a lot of work and there are the decisions about feeding, perhaps on a train or aeroplane, and wondering how a new place or even the water will affect the baby. Only some kinds of bottled water are suitable. Ask your health professionals for advice about this. Breastmilk is obviously the safest drink. As you take off and land at an airport, the pressure changes can cause pain in a baby's ears. As she does not understand the need to swallow, you can offer the nice surprise of a quick feed to encourage this.

Different cultures react to breastfeeding in all kinds of different ways and you may find it easier to feed in public in some European countries. If you are still breastfeeding at all and are going abroad, it is probably well worth keeping up even just one breastfeed to maintain one stable element in the baby's pattern of the day.

Starting on other foods

As you continue to feed, the question of adding different foods will come up from advisors, or from your own response to the baby. Solids had been offered at a wide variety of ages during this century, as late as nine months and as early as two weeks. Worldwide, there are many forbidden foods for babies, but also a lot of just giving the baby a bit of what the family is eating either straight or pre-chewed. Many grandparents may feel quite happy about little tastes of egg, wheat based rusks, and so on as early as six weeks – food which we now feel are the very ones most likely to lead to early sensitising of the baby to 'foreign' proteins.

There is a good deal of information available about this from your health visitor, and there are leaflets such as the ones from the Health Education Authority and the NCT. Commercially sponsored leaflets, of course, tend – however subtly – to advertise their own products and may be quite keen for you to see tins, jars and packets as an important part of your baby's diet from an early age. Your health professional will probably confirm that it is wise to introduce other foods very slowly, a little at a time, and to remember that milk will be the main food for your baby until she is at least a year old. You can watch for reactions to a particular food like tummy pain, wheezing, runny nose, sore eyes, or rashes.

When to start

The Department of Health recommends starting to offer solids when your baby is between four and six months old. At around three months there is often a growth spurt, so it is worth trying the usual two days or so of responsive feeding before rushing into giving solid food. A baby who can hold things and is able to sit up a little is showing signs of being ready. It may help to ask yourself if you are beginning to feel uncomfortable with the baby watching every mouthful of your food as it goes from plate to mouth, or even making a grab for what you are eating. If this is happening, it is a sign that she will probably be interested in starting on her own exploration of different tastes.

Offering extra food is sometimes seen as very much a part of the weaning process and if you were really enjoying breastfeeding, it can feel a little threatening.

'I am quite disappointed now he takes more solids, that he wants less from me.'

Inevitably, the proportion of breastmilk in the diet will fall slightly because of the new 'solids' (they are not very solid at all at this time, of course). In fact, the baby will still need milk for many months, and most mothers find they easily combine feeding on the breast with a baby's progression from stewed apple and baby rice to finger foods like raw carrot pieces or casserole without the salt. If a health visitor's quick reference to starting the baby on a bit of baby rice leaves you feeling your milk is regarded as being insufficient, do find out if she meant this. You may find that she simply thought you might like to get the baby used to taking things off a spoon as she was reaching out so well for things now.

You may see it as a new and exciting discovery for the baby or just something you feel you have to do. One agreed medical reason for offering some extra food by six months is that the baby's iron stores, in her liver since she was in the womb, begin to run out at around this time and that a baby who does not begin to taste and chew food at the stage where she is ready, may find it more difficult to accept it later. You could ask for an iron test from your GP if you feel under pressure and the baby seems quite unwilling to cooperate. Someone else may find it easier to start the baby on other food. After all, she has come to expect only milk from you.

What to give

If the baby seems ready, sloppy baby rice, mixed with your own milk for a familiar taste, or puréed apple, carrot or other fruit or vegetable, can be offered after a breastfeed, at first in tiny amounts. If you are trying to avoid cow's milk for some reason, read the packets very carefully as many manufacturers now add dried milk to the baby rice. Put a little bit on a spoon and see if the baby is interested in sucking it off. From six months easy foods are sieved cottage cheese, yoghurts, soups and so on. If there are allergies in the family it is worth avoiding milk products until later in the first year, and it is also a good idea not to eat peanuts yourself while you are breastfeeding. Avoid salt, sugar, or too many spices. Honey is not safe for babies either. If you are a vegetarian you will be giving a lot of thought to food values anyway, and know for example that sources of iron other than meat, such as apricots, are possible. The vegetarian and vegan societies produce useful information (see page 202).

How to give it

Some babies object quite strongly to being spoonfed with thin mixtures, but at around eight months they may quite happily pick up pieces of banana, apple, or celery sticks to gnaw on, or hard baked bread fingers smeared with various suitably spready things while you are eating. In this way they will be very happy to join in with your meal. Obviously you need to stay around while babies are eating anything solid and lumpy ready to turn them upside down, and slap them around the shoulder blade if necessary, to dislodge a misplaced cube of pineapple or a piece of cheese.

When you begin solid food, the baby's motions will begin to become darker and more solid. Many foods, such as carrots come out in the motions still looking pretty much like they went in all through toddlerhood. The useful vitamins and so on have been used but the toddler's digestion cannot yet cope with the cellulose.

Long-term breastfeeding

As the journey goes on, it may again be especially important to have the support of other mothers if you are feeding beyond the first year or so. 'Breast is best – as long as you only do it for six months' seemed to be the message I was getting.' If in the end you decide that continuing feeding is what you, the baby and others are happy with – perhaps well into the second or third years – then you may encounter some social pressures and need support. You may begin to think about ways of limiting the accessibility of your breasts to the baby in public places, and finding words for feeding which do not embarrass you. 'By now I knew quite a few other women feeding toddlers and my confidence in the idea had grown . . . my friends had grown used to the sight of us feeding, but new acquaintances looked a bit dumbfounded.'

'I was also given some appalling advice from my doctor such as "Are you still only breastfeeding?" at six weeks.'

Avoiding another pregnancy

While you are breastfeeding a tiny baby often during the day and night, you are less likely to conceive another child, but if the baby has an extra long sleep, it can lead to a fall in your hormones, so allowing you to ovulate and become fertile. Your likelihood of conception is related to a whole series of things, like your personal hormone levels, how well you are eating, how frequently and how long the baby is feeding, and so on. Together with your partner, you do need to consider whether or not to avoid another pregnancy, and decide about contraception. Your GP or Family Planning Association Clinic will be a source of information. Basically, your choices are between the contraceptive pill and barrier methods. The combined pill which contains oestrogen is not recommended for breastfeeding mothers since it affects milk supply. The mini-pill is often prescribed for breastfeeding mothers as the one synthetic hormone it contains theoretically has no effect on milk supply, although it does pass into the milk. However, all women are individuals, and no studies have been carried out which show for certain that milk supply remains unaffected. In practice some mothers who begin taking the mini-pill earlier than about six weeks do notice that there is a slight fall in the milk supply, but if they persevere, feeding more often for a while, the baby seems to adjust the supply back to the right amount. It may be that starting the pill coincides with one of the baby's growth spurts, or possibly that the slightly different taste of the milk while the pill is being taken makes the baby less enthusiastic to feed and so leads to her taking less at first and a build-up of milk supplies. It is possible to see whether the mini-pill has any effect on your milk supply and find another method of contraception if it does. Contraceptive injections, which may have a similar effect, are impossible to reverse for three months.

Since it is very difficult to know the long-term effects on a baby of even small amounts of extra hormones in the mother's milk, some women prefer to delay chemical contraception until the baby is weaned.

Being pregnant

If you become pregnant while you are still breastfeeding, you may wonder whether to wean or not. There is no rush to decide, as breastfeeding is not at all likely to harm the baby growing inside you. The only times to worry would be if you were experiencing any pain or bleeding, or have a history of delivering prematurely. If you are being very sick, you may feel you cannot keep down enough food for the three of you. If the usual nipple tenderness at the beginning of pregnancy makes you very sore it may help to get the milk supply going before the baby takes the breast.

You may be worried that your toddler will feel pushed out if weaned suddenly.

It will seem a long way away to falling in love with a new baby, deciding whose needs count most and what is a genuine need as opposed to a habit – if it is possible to make such a distinction. You need also to include your own needs in any decision. As pregnancy goes on, you may find practical problems like the disappearance of your lap means the baby has to feed lying beside you, or standing up, if he is old enough. The older baby may find that the milk supply falls as the new baby gets nearer to being born and feel it is not worth going on, and he may not like the new taste of the colostrum ready for the next baby. If your previous child is still needing a lot of milk for his nutrition, then you might need to consider complementing your own milk with formula. It is quite possible to continue breastfeeding past the birth of your next baby, offering her the colostrum made for her, as well as giving the first child a chance at feeding.

'I fed my first child all the way through my pregnancy, with no problems at all, and then "tandem fed" them both till the younger one stopped. None of this was planned and I started out with no strong idea or thought upon the matter at all. It just seemed to be what felt right at the time . . . nor do I feel any more tired now than I would expect to be as a mother of two normal toddlers!'

Chapter Nine

Overcoming crises

'Immediately he was admitted to hospital he was put on a ventilator . . . there followed approximately 12 weeks of expressing milk so that he could be fed minute amounts through a naso-gastric tube. I wonder how I managed to retain the will to do it, but because he was sedated it was the only thing I could do for him.'

There are so many new experiences when first becoming a mother that each one can seem like a mini-crisis. Where a quick trip to the supermarket, or swimming, or even a holiday used to be simple to organise, such outings can now feel rather worrying. Problems which actually concern the mother's breasts or the baby's feeding behaviour are dealt with in Chapter 10, but in this chapter the rest of life is the subject matter, for it heavily influences breastfeeding.

Bumps or turns in the road may confuse the breastfeeding mother, from the christening and its party to opening the door to find a parent you last saw ten years ago on your doorstep. Some need practical strategies, and all have varying emotional repercussions. Each mother, in each family situation, reacts differently, and every new turn teaches you how to cope.

Events

'He was just six weeks old and I had arranged to have the christening the week before Christmas . . . a bevvy of relations descended and began to tell me that all this organising would be affecting my milk supply, just what you want to hear when your milk is the sole source of nourishment . . . despite all these things my little boy continued to thrive and put on weight.'

Moving house, being without water for a day, and so on, all bring lots of planning and work. You may find you are worrying about worrying, thinking it will do something to your milk supply. It can help to remember that it is not the work, or the worrying, which may temporarily diminish your milk, but the time the baby spends being cuddled and jiggled by others, or being left to cry, when you know she wants feeding. If you are very anxious, with people making life stressful, it is just possible that your milk may take a little longer than usual to let down. You can explain the situation to the baby and wait together with her, perhaps sighing out the tension as feeding itself calms you.

Crises

Crises may include family disasters and worries, from real or threatened redundancy and financial concerns to arguments, or even something upsetting on the news. Women have never been insulated from these aspects of life. Breastfeeding can continue, perhaps as a calm amid the storm, especially if you can find someone to talk about the concerns with.

The death of a relative brings practical disruption of a high level, with the need to attend a funeral and sort out belongings. If the person dying is someone very close, such as your own mother, an especially loved grandmother, or sister, you may be so upset that you feel you cannot carry on feeding the baby. People may tell you that the shock will take away your milk. This is not at all likely, and you may find that although you are very upset,

---

'I was very anxious that it should work . . . this added to the tensions at home where my husband was trying to adjust to the new happenings and had his own work problems.'

sitting down to feed the baby is a great reassurance that life, love and nurturing continue despite great sadness and loss, as perhaps the person who has died would have wished it to do. 'My mother (my best friend) died early in my pregnancy. I couldn't talk to my mother-in-law, so all my decisions (and panics) had to be my own or talked through with my friend from hospital.'

If you have lost someone close before the birth of the baby, grief can return as you remember what it would have been like to show the baby to them. It is hard to rejoice in a new life while needing to take time to mourn.

Illness

In the baby

If your baby becomes ill, even with something as trivial as a cold, feeding is the first thing to be affected. She may be hot and floppy and want to sleep off her infection, or she may want much more frequent feeds to make her feel more comfortable. These feeds are likely to be shorter than usual, as she may well only want to have foremilk to quench her thirst and not feel like 'eating' creamy hindmilk. This can lower your milk supply and leave you a bit unprepared for her new healthy appetite once she feels better. The effect of her regained enthusiasm for your milk feels rather like a growth spurt and you need to be ready to feed a lot for a while.

Older babies who are not well may refuse other food and return only to the breast. It is now known that this is the best cure for tummy bugs.

In the mother

It can be frightening at the best of times to be ill, but when you also feel responsible for nourishing a baby it can be very worrying. If you are a single parent it may be best to go to a friend or relative to be cared for or ask someone to come to look after you and the baby at home. The person looking after you could bring the baby for feeding and you could stay lying down to offer the breast. 'I had the 'flu for a month on and off and carried on feeding even when quite feverish.'

If you find it impossible to feed, the bottom line is that some way of feeding even a baby who has steadfastly refused a bottle so far *can* be found. Try a spoon at first, a sturdy eggcup by three months or so, and later a beaker. If you have diarrhoea or vomiting, people may tell you your milk will go, but even if you are only able to keep sipping water, your body will make manufacturing breastmilk a priority. The baby may want to feed very frequently as they do in places where mothers are regularly poorly nourished. The supply will build itself again. If you feel you cannot bear the stress of your baby's frequent feeds and someone else bottle-feeds her for a while, the milk can be called back (see Relactation on page 175).

If you become ill with a contagious or infectious disease, you may worry, especially if the baby is young. You will already, however, have exposed the baby to the virus or bacteria responsible some time before you realised you were ill, so removing yourself may do little to prevent the baby from getting it. Ask your doctor whether useful precautions can be taken to minimise infection for each different illness – for example, in chicken pox you can avoid letting the baby touch any weeping areas. It is good though to remember that while you were developing the disease, your body was manufacturing antibodies to it, which will already be passing into the baby through your milk. This means that if the baby does catch whatever you have, the effect may be less severe than if you had not been breastfeeding, and you can continue to offer comfort as well as food while she is ill.

Hospitalisation of another child

'. . . the great comfort I experienced at being able to feed my six-weeks-old baby when my daughter was admitted to hospital, seriously ill. Thanks to the kindness of the nursing staff who provided a cot in the intensive care unit, I was able to stay with my daughter until she recovered and to continue breastfeeding my baby too.'

If an elder child should have to go into hospital for a while, it is nearly always possible to take the baby into hospital with you so that breastfeeding can continue. However, if for example there were to be whooping cough or other unpleasant diseases on the ward, you might feel better if your partner went with the older child.

Hospitalisation of the baby

Some babies will at some point need to be in hospital for a while, perhaps for tests or because of a birth defect which needs surgery. It is particularly difficult if your baby needs hospital treatment in a paediatric unit while you are struggling to get breastfeeding going. You may need to rely especially on someone with a good knowledge of breastfeeding, or to ask for a midwife to visit you or to get in touch with a breastfeeding counsellor. If a baby is suddenly admitted, you may find your milk supply is affected by the separation, but it will return, when the baby needs you most. You may not be able to offer it directly, though, and may have to express (see page 156) to keep up the supply and to stop yourself from getting blocked ducts. If your child is under five years old you have a right to stay with her. Before operations there is generally a fasting time of up to eight hours, but you may be able to persuade medical staff that as breastmilk stays a much shorter time in a baby's stomach, this need not be so long. Afterwards, drips or traction may make breastfeeding quite hard practically, and you will need to ask the nurses for guidance.

If you are in hospital

'Panic – could it be an abscess? . . . Spend sleepless nights worrying whether may have to go into hospital – who would look after baby? How would he be fed? How would we mange? . . . Discovered later that babies can be accommodated in hospital with sick mum. Wish I'd known earlier.'

This is perhaps one of the greatest fears for breastfeeding mothers. If you are the one to need treatment and you cannot speak for yourself someone else needs to explain to the hospital staff that you are still breastfeeding, and that not only does your baby need your milk, but your breasts need expressing so that you will not add to your problems by overfull breasts.

Many situations involving hospitalisation do not mean the end of breastfeeding, although there may be some disruption to normal patterns. Most tests have little effect and X-rays do not harm milk, but some diagnosis using radioactive material means stopping feeding for a while. Ask about this. If your hospitalisation is planned, this gives you time to ask about anaesthetics to be used. In case it is felt that milk affected by anaesthetics or pain relief may need to be expressed and thrown away, you can build up a supply of expressed milk in a freezer in advance. You could take in a hand pump in a steriliser with you, or hire a larger pump (see page 158).

If you have been able to obtain the agreement of a consultant to taking the baby with you on to the ward, it may be as well to check with the ward sister before you go that you are both expected.

Any drug treatment will obviously lead to you asking a lot of questions, as circumstances, such as the age of the baby, can change things. It may be possible to give quite powerful drugs as long as the baby is monitored, or alternatives which do not affect the baby may be prescribed. It is worth getting in touch with a breastfeeding counsellor for although she has not the specialist medical knowledge herself to help, she has access to someone who may be able to. She can also help you think around your concern, and perhaps help you to focus on good questions to ask. It will also probably help your distress to speak to someone who understands how strongly you feel about the issue. She may be able to put you in touch with someone from a local or nationally held 'special situations register', possibly containing people who have had similar experiences.

Making decisions

As in all crises, it is best to be able to talk, think and wait, rather than be rushed or decide at the last minute what you want to do. Try to find ways of buying time so that you are able to explore your options properly and bear in mind that even an interrupted lactation can often be resumed with support. As with getting help initially, it will make you more sure in the end that all was done to protect your breastfeeding if you find out as much as you can of the implications of any illness, and its treatment.

Sudden endings

If your baby dies you will be surrounded by things which remind you of her, but one of the saddest things is the way that your breasts continue for a while to make milk. Expressing as little as you can to make your breasts feel comfortable will help. The doctor can offer tablets for pain relief, hormone type drugs to reduce milk supply and diuretics which reduce fluid in your body. A well-fitting bra may help. Talking and talking about your baby will do the most to help you and your partner, and a breastfeeding counsellor can help here if you want one.

Worrying

Of course, it is only a few women or babies who need to go into hospital during the breastfeeding period, and many of these situations are very unlikely to happen to you. If you find you are constantly thinking about this kind of problem rather than enjoying your baby, talk to your health visitor or doctor.

CHAPTER TEN

Overcoming problems

> '*Most people who knew me would say that I fed successfully and my daughter thrived. Yet I found the normal experience of breastfeeding painful.*'

Breastfeeding is a subjective experience: 'I got very sore and cracked nipples, the usual things, but the whole experience has been wonderful.'

Feeling that things are going wrong and having your worries dismissed can be upsetting. Breastfeeding problems can make you feel very low indeed, and can seem to spoil what you may feel ought to be a happy time.

> '*He'd lost 4oz. At last I was believed. There was a problem.*'

Equally, if you had a good start, or fed very happily last time, the first snag can seem quite a hurdle. If you have more than one problem, or the same trouble keeps coming back, it is even worse.

> '*By now I felt as if life had stopped completely and I was just a milking machine. I was not too keen on this baby either who had given me a big scar, sore nipples, sleepless nights etc. I could not seem to cope with everyday things at all.*'

This mother, ill with mastitis, did eventually stop breastfeeding. Like her, if you find that the problems you encounter are too much for you, then Chapter 13 on stopping may be of some help.

Our reactions to difficulties vary a lot: indeed many mothers find they can be helped and go on to enjoy breastfeeding again. Getting competent help is obviously vital. If breastfeeding hurts, there must be something wrong. Understanding what may be happening can be a first step, so in this chapter all the dismal side of breastfeeding, which many women never experience, is gathered for close scrutiny.

Is there enough milk?

This is probably the most common concern of breastfeeding mothers. You know that you can tell if the baby is getting enough by her seven or eight wet terry nappies a day, or several disposables heavy with urine, and her 'scrambled egg' motions. On average, the baby's growth rate needs to be keeping up with what is expected on the charts at the clinic, bearing in mind that breast-fed babies do not all grow at the same rate. Your health visitor will be the obvious person to talk to about the baby's weight.

If you are concerned that your baby isn't getting enough milk, you can also look at her behaviour. Is she normally alert and not too pale? Does she ask for feeds at least six times a day if she is not yet eating much solid food?

Just occasionally 'polite' babies do not tell you they are hungry: 'he would fall asleep after sucking for a few minutes and I would assume he had fed enough and put him back in the pram . . . ' They have learnt to conserve energy by not crying. This is quite unusual, of course, as most babies will not let you forget to feed them. Once they have had enough food to realise how nice milk is, they can catch up in a big way: 'then we had all the long, frequent feeds to build up the milk supply, but from then on I actually enjoyed feeding him and welcomed the chance to sit down and relax.'

What if there isn't enough?

If your baby is not growing well, or is never settled on the breast or afterwards, there are various things to try before you turn to complementary bottle feeds, or change to formula altogether. If you can, discuss all your options with a health professional or breastfeeding counsellor before you do anything.

'My health visitor advised feeding him two-and-a-half-to-three-hourly and topping him up with 1–2oz formula after feeds if he was still not settled, and not let him feed for more than 30 minutes. This helped in the short term, but I do not think it helped my milk supply.'

First you need to look again to see if the baby is well enough attached to the breast to be getting a satisfying feed – does she ever spit you out as if she can't take another drop for example, or does she always stay on the breast until you have to take her off? Does she come to the breast with her mouth wide open, her lips turned out, and her chin close to the breast?: 'he never seemed to open his mouth wide enough to latch on, as the books said he should.' Listen for the sounds of soft gulping as let-down happens. If this is not what you find, seek help with positioning. If you have done all this, yet the baby is still growing too slowly, ask the doctor to check there is not a hidden problem which can slow down the baby's growth, such as an infection.

You know that feeding more often will help too, and that it is well worth letting the baby stay on the first breast to reach the hindmilk she wants before offering the other side. Remembering to look after yourself will also help. The NCT produces a leaflet about making more milk which you may find helpful (see Useful Reading). It is a good idea to look back again at the positioning section on pages 25–34 and the section which looks at signs which people often interpret as meaning there is not enough milk on page 109.

Getting rid of complementary bottles

If you have been using top-up feeds, you may feel you have been rushed into them too quickly. You may have started with just one small feed, and now see them spreading and becoming more acceptable to your baby. If you are giving more than a few

Ways to help build up your milk supply

- offer the breast first
- cut down the number of complementary feeds and replace a bottle with a cup
- reduce the amount of formula
- if you cannot persuade the baby to go on feeding for long, try expressing your own milk to give
- offer only small bottle feeds so the baby does not sleep for too long
- use a teat with smaller holes
- encourage the baby to wait a few minutes before offering the complement
- put the baby back to the breast afterwards if she will cooperate

Encouraging signs

- the baby's motions may become less solid and more yellow
- a baby takes more milk from you each week (until you being to give serious amounts of semi-solid food)
- you may begin to experience fuller breasts again.

So if you are managing to hold the complements steady, your own personal milk supply is actually increasing. This means you are responding to your baby's needs and it is likely you can extend this response to meet her full needs in time.

ounces a day, it would be unwise suddenly to withdraw them altogether, but there are many ways of cutting them down while you work on building up your own milk supply: '. . . supplementing need not be the end of breastfeeding . . . I built up the milk once the soreness had gone by more frequent feeding.' Getting information and support while you do this will be helpful, so ringing a breastfeeding counsellor will be a good move.

If you are totally bottle-feeding, yet would like to start breastfeeding again, it may help to look at the section on Relactation on page 175.

Getting milk into proportion

As well as filling the baby up with two drinks, giving two feeds of foremilk from both breasts can lead to what is usually called 'colic', as there can be to much milk-sugar for the baby to cope with in such a large – but not very satisfying – feed. The baby may cry in pain, pull off the breast while feeding, and have green motions. Let the baby decide about staying on the breast.

Too much milk?

'People said I was lucky to have plenty of milk but I hated it!' The baby may find this hard too, so you could try a semi-upright position for her. In desperation, you can feed lying on your back with the baby on your tummy for a while. You may have to hold her forehead up while she is still too young to do this for herself.

In the long term, you may find it especially useful to make sure that the baby does not get two lots of foremilk, and, if she is satisfied with this, encourage her to take one side only each feed for a while. You could try coming back twice to the same breast during a time when you expect a period of closely spaced feeds, such as many babies have in the evening.

Mothers and milk

If you are still leaking a lot, some of the above section may help. So may splashing the nipples with cold water night and morning. A clean, man-sized handkerchief, or one-way nappy liners may help. If milk drips from the 'other' breast during feeds it is possible to use sterilised plastic drip catchers inside the bra so as not to waste it – useful for freezing if you intend going out or returning to work. Be careful they do not press into your breast too much. Whatever they do, some mothers go on making a surplus.

To stop the let-down if it begins, you can fold your arms and press backwards against your breasts for a few seconds. Dark and patterned clothes may help you. If leaking worries you, talk to someone. Sometimes you may suddenly feel very full of milk if the baby sleeps through the night, or feeds less because of a cold or whatever. Simply expressing a little bit should help, or you can wake the baby, or try feeding her asleep – even if it is only just enough to get your milk flowing. One rather strange remedy is to apply cold raw cabbage leaves inside your bra until they are warm. They seem to 'draw' the heat and discomfort from the breasts. The NCT produces a leaflet called *Too Much Milk* (see page 198).

Sore nipples

If you have had soreness at the beginning of feeding and it has passed, and then it happens again with sore and pink skin which feels rough, this may be thrush of the nipple. Thrush is on our skin all the time, but is not usually a nuisance. It may appear after a course of antibiotics. If you are suffering from it the baby may be affected too – look for white spots which will not easily rub off in her mouth or throat, bulky motions, or a sore bottom. She may not show any symptoms. Your GP can give good treatment, drops for the baby, and cream for you: it may help to suggest that you think the two conditions may be related. It is important that you are both treated, even if the baby shows no signs, and that you go on taking the treatment for ten to 14 days even if the symptoms go away sooner. Meanwhile, to discourage the thrush, at each feed you can use a teaspoonful of bicarbonate of soda in a cup of warm water as a wash for your nipple area and the baby's mouth. But avoid using this for more than a few days as it contains salt. Dummies and teats can carry thrush too, and need to be sterilised by boiling for 20 minutes if there is a problem.

It appears to be possible for thrush to spread into the ducts of the breast, with deep pains which are felt particularly after a feed. It is possible to treat this too. If you keep getting thrush it may be that it is in your vagina, and your partner may need treatment too. There are oral treatments for thrush of the ducts. A very good leaflet about thrush is available from the Breastfeeding Network (address on page 203). This is another area where it can be helpful to talk to a breastfeeding counsellor.

There are other causes for soreness apart from thrush, which you may like to consult your doctor about – dermatitis can be caused in some people by coming into contact with detergents, and eczema is possible on nipples too: 'I had eczema on my nipples before and during pregnancy but with the use of steroid creams I cleared it in time.' One mother with quite severe eczema found breastfeeding surprisingly painfree despite concern from health professionals. If you use hydrocortizone cream to clear up eczema it will need to be washed off before each feed. Teething babies may produce very acidic saliva which 'burns' the mother. It may help to wash it off after feeds if this is a problem. In cold weather, poor circulation can cause some mothers, usually those who have fingers and toes that turn white in cold weather, to experience painful nipples which turn white as the baby feeds. Warmth is an obvious answer and a cup of tea may help as it contains a chemical which opens up small blood vessels.

Blocked ducts

These may feel like uncomfortably tender lumps, and are caused by milk building up like a traffic jam behind a temporary obstruction, such as a bra strap or arm – yours or the baby's during feeding or sleeping. You can help yourself by feeding first from that side, leaning over the baby if possible, letting the baby's chin be nearest to the blockage if you can, and massaging gently as you do so and at other times. You can use a soapy wide-toothed comb, stroking gently towards the nipple to break up the blockage.

Later, a small piece of milk solid may emerge as a little white spot through an opening on the nipple. You can help it out by expressing, warmth – especially in a bath – and even a sterilised needle. Someone else using a pump while you massage your breast by hand may double the effectiveness. There are conditions which cause more long-lasting lumps, most of which are harmless, but if any lump does not go away and causes you concern, whether it is painful or not, your GP is able to refer you to a specialist. It is not enough to accept reassurance that all is probably well, even from an experienced GP.

Mastitis

Perhaps the most important piece of information regarding mastitis is that there is no need to stop feeding if you have it. If you get a blocked duct or mastitis it is important to check that your baby is well attached to your breast while feeding, as it is likely that leaving milk in a part of the breast can cause these conditions and that draining the breast well can both prevent them and help in their cure.

Mastitis means inflammation of the breast, and if you are suffering from it you would notice a red sore patch and begin to feel ill, as if you had 'flu, and many women feel tearful as well. This may be because you have picked up an infection which has gone into the milk ducts or breast tissue, or it may just be that you have had a blocked duct which has leaked out milk into the breast. When this happens, the breast reacts strongly to either the infection or the milk in the wrong place, rushing a blood supply to it to take it away – hence the red patch. For the infection, you need antibiotics; for the milk in the wrong place, you do not. Unfortunately, without counting how many bacteria there are in the milk, no one can know which type of problem it is, and it is not a good idea to wait to find out for too long, since an untreated infection could lead to an abscess. In any case, leaking into the tissue may lead to an infection. So most mothers make an appointment to see the doctor on the same day. Some doctors and midwives now understand that it may be possible to avoid the use of antibiotics in mastitis unless other treatments prove ineffective, and suggest that you use an anti-inflammatory drug such as ibuprofen instead, while making sure the breast is drained as comfortably as possible.*

Meanwhile, there is a lot which you can do to try to clear the mastitis yourself. Feeding the baby on the sore side first, leaking into a warm bath or using a bowl or flannels to warm the breasts may help a lot. If you are able to feed the baby while your breast is hanging down this may be particularly helpful: you can put the baby on the floor or a coffee table. Gentle massage or expressing will help, and cold compresses after a feed to calm everything down. Moving the arm on the same side will help the blood supply to deal with the problem, but you need also to get plenty of rest if you feel ill.

If after working at this you feel an improvement you could always cancel the appointment, or go to show the doctor what is happening, or even discuss with him or her whether it might be a good idea to have a prescription for antibiotic, but perhaps not take the course if the improvement continues. If you do begin the course of antibiotics, you have to finish it and you may find this gives the baby some diarrhoea. This will not harm her in the long term but she will probably want longer feeds which may also help your breasts to be cleared out. Many women eat yoghurt while they are on antibiotics to encourage the good bacteria in their bodies – the ones which destroy thrush and help us to digest our food well.

If you find mastitis is a problem more than once here are some suggestions:

- check the baby's positioning in case one part of the breast is being neglected
- make sure your fingers are not pressing into the breast tissue as you feed
- avoid too much animal fat
- stop using any creams
- cut down on tea, coffee, cola (even avoid caffeine completely for a while) and any cigarettes
- eat well
- ask the doctor to take a culture of milk to see if a more appropriate antibiotic might be necessary – or a longer course
- ask for a swab from the baby's throat and nose in case she keeps giving you an infection

You may already have experience of homeopathy or aromatherapy as alternative forms of treatment in other circumstances. There are alternative treatments available for mastitis as for other conditions. It is best to go to a practitioner who is properly qualified in his or her field for help.

Abscesses

These happen to very few breastfeeding mothers. They generally come after mastitis, although they can just flare up as a sudden infection. They are soft, pus-filled lumps which may not feel as painful as a blocked duct. You may well feel very ill though. The baby will not be harmed by any blood or pus coming out of the nipple and will just be sick if there is too much to cope with. The

Royal College of Midwives believes that during treatment, breastfeeding should continue as it speeds healing, but sometimes antibiotics which are incompatible with breastfeeding are prescribed. This treatment can be enough on its own, but often an abscess needs draining either surgically or by using a syringe several times to draw out its contents. This second treatment is more recent and avoids a general anaesthetic, spending a night in hospital, or having a wound which needs to be dressed. Nevertheless, antibiotics would be given for a few weeks. If there is a wound which is slow to heal, it is possible to allow the supply on the affected side to dwindle by gradually feeding less, and then build it up later.

Other breast lumps

'When I was six-seven months a bean-sized lump developed in my left breast which my doctor thought was probably a blocked duct . . . eight days after the birth the area around the lump became pink/red and it started throbbing. I felt fluey – mastitis. I was given antibiotics . . . the lump remained . . . a month after the birth I saw a consultant and a sample was taken which confirmed the lump was benign . . . gradually the lump got smaller and disappeared.'

During breastfeeding, it is possible for women to find lumps which are usually cysts in their breasts. Most will turn out to be harmless (they are sometimes filled with milk), and fade away, but any lump which remains should be shown to your GP, and you may feel you need proper reassurance that you haven't got cancer.

Babies

All kinds of things can upset the way a baby feeds, and that can distress you: 'baby throws a wobbly after a long car journey and refuses all feeds for eight hours. I get hysterical.' Lots of visitors and cuddling may disrupt things for a day or so; even breast-feeding babies pick up illnesses. If your baby is floppy, hot, coughing or obviously in pain with screaming fits, you will want to take her to the doctor. Earache, a urinary infection, even the aftermath of injections, can disrupt the feeding pattern which may be beginning to emerge. Holding a bunged-up baby upright for a while before a feed and getting her to sneeze by tickling her nose with a tiny wisp of cotton wool may help. Also, the doctor can prescribe nose drops.

Tummy bugs

Diarrhoea is smelly and there may be 12 motions or more a day. If the baby is not ill but just has one or two green stools this is more likely to be caused by too much foremilk or something you ate. If the baby is ill and being sick you will obviously want to see the doctor, as you will if the baby is doing regular projectile vomiting which goes a long distance across the room. It may help to make a diagnosis if you are able to feed the baby while the doctor feels her stomach. This would show the extent of the problem and help show if it is one which can be put right with a fairly small operation.

Often babies who are ill sleep a lot, or have many little drinks of foremilk which keep them comforted, cool them down, and replace fluid lost by fever, diarrhoea or vomiting.* If your baby feeds less for a day or so, your milk supply will drop to match her needs. If you are feeling uncomfortable, express a little milk. But if you want to keep a tip-top supply going, then you can express more and freeze it ready for later if you need it anytime. If the illness is more long-lasting, then you need to keep expressing in mind as a way to maintain your milk supply. Otherwise do not be surprised if your baby begins to be extra hungry when she is feeling better. Not only does she need to make up for nutrition not taken while she was off-colour, but she has not been able to stimulate your breasts in the usual way to make balanced meals, so she will feed long and hard and often. Remembering that it took a couple of days for the supply to reduce to match her needs, will help you to cope over the next period as she works up your milk supply again.

Teething

Teething can cause pain in the mouth, and more saliva to be made. Sometimes this gives the baby a lot of extra motions for a few days.

If a baby has pain in her mouth she may bite down on anything to try to relieve it, including your breast. Taking the baby off the breast as you say 'no' usually works: 'He has five teeth and has only tried to bite me twice. A firm no stopped him immediately.' This is most likely to happen at the beginnings and ends of feeds. It may help to get the milk flowing first, and to stop feeding as soon as the baby is no longer taking a swallow with every suck. Offering alternative chewing may help. Try teething rings which can be put in the fridge to cool her gums down, or finger food before feeds if the baby is old enough.

Refusing to feed

Sometimes babies refuse to feed and it can happen on one side alone or both sides.

'I am sure there was never as much milk on that side . . . she had reached the stage when she realised that she could have some control over events . . . offering her the least favoured side first just meant that she worked herself up into such a state that it was a real trial to get her to feed at all.'

If the baby misses more than a couple of feeds, it is wise to begin to offer breastmilk on a spoon, and watch for listlessness, dry nappies, and a dry mouth which may be signs of dehydration, and seek medical help if you are worried. Express milk to keep the supply going.

Babies may refuse the breast if they have had a shock, for example if they bit you and your reaction was to drop them or shout, or they simply choked hard on a lot of milk. There are many ways to get round this but it is not a good idea to force the issue. If the baby refuses one side only, it is fine to offer the other,

Possible reasons for refusing to feed

- a big bowel movement on the way
- teething, or the pain of thrush
- let-down being a little slow
- earache or tummy ache when she feeds
- the milk tasting different – perhaps garlic, if she is not used to it. Food eaten takes roughly 8 to 12 hours to come through into your milk and about 24 hours to stop affecting the baby.
- milk during and after mastitis tasting saltier
- one antibiotic, flagyl, tasting bitter in the milk
- milk tasting odd immediately after exercise or around the time of a period

and then gently slide her across but this may not work after six weeks old. If you find nothing works, remember that a baby can perfectly well be fed from one side only.

If she refuses both sides, she may feed in the bath, or when she is sleepy or asleep, in a dark room or swaddled. Mothers often instinctively try standing and singing or humming while rocking. Express a little milk first if the flow is overwhelming, or if you feel the let-down might have been slow.

If she continues to refuse to feed, it can help to avoid breast-feeding for a day or so and offer spoons or cups. But do give her lots of cuddles and skin-to-skin contact, avoiding the usual breastfeeding position and wait for the baby to make the first move. If the baby is over six months, you may decide that she is weaning herself. If you were not ready for this, it is no use other people telling you it is all right. You may like to read Chapter 13 on Stopping.

If you are worried because you need to give bottles and they are being refused see Chapter 11 on Working and Feeding.

Colic

There is very little agreement about what colic is or even if it exists, but some babies do seem to get a lot of wind and tummy-

'I think the feeling of guilt was the hardest to cope with – I constantly analysed what I was eating and wondered whether anything could have upset him.'

ache, and it may help to try different ways of easing it. You may, for example, like to try:

- avoiding too much foremilk
- putting the baby on your shoulder, or between your knees and rubbing her back
- making sure the baby gets as much hindmilk as she wants – if she is still feeding all evening, when colic is often at its worst, try returning to the same breast (once or twice) instead of switching over
- gently lifting the baby with your arms round her ribcage and letting her legs dangle
- putting a hot water bottle in the cot – take it out before the baby gets in
- a warm deep bath together
- cutting out 'suspicious' foods – things which you either find upset you or you really like
- avoiding too much coffee, tea and chocolate – they can make a baby irritable
- give up smoking
- as a last resort you might think about trying a week without cow's milk products (see page 126)

When a baby is 'fighting' the breast, it is hard not to feel very hurt and rejected, as if the little flailing fists were deliberately pushing you away. But remember that for months, the baby does not even recognise you as a separate person, so cannot hate you – she just feels pain when she feeds, yet wants to eat and drink and so is very unhappy and confused about what to do. Some parents have found their babies with colic have benefited from a course of cranial osteopathy with a qualified practitioner. In this treatment the baby's head and neck are very gently manipulated to put right any damage done at birth. This may be especially helpful where the baby is unhappy a lot of the time and had a very quick entry into the world or an assisted delivery.

Medical help

For many of these problems you will be turning to your GP for medical help. No one complains when this is perfectly adequate and given with compassion, and mostly this is the case. But it is important to find out why anyone feels you should do something that you are not happy about, like stopping feeding, or offering complementary feeds. It may be that there are assumptions being made about breastfeeding, or you, which you would like the chance to talk about some more. Suppose, for example, you developed mastitis when your baby was eight months old. Feeling ill and in pain you may not realise what the GP has said to you until you are back at home and just about to take the prescription.

'As I walked out of his surgery his parting shot was "By the way don't feed the baby while taking this antibiotic." He gave me no advice as to what to do at all . . . I felt that I had two lumps of concrete stuck in front of me.'

You might find it useful to discuss your options with your health visitor or breastfeeding counsellor, or to ring and explain to the doctor how you feel about breastfeeding, if you did not feel well enough at the time to explain. Going with your partner or a friend may help with this.

Obviously, some women avoid the issue by seeing a different doctor next time, but this means you may lose the chance to build up a good relationship with your own GP. If your doctor is prescribing for you do remind him that you are still feeding even if this means telling him you are carrying on when he has suggested you stop.

Obviously, every problem and difficult situation cannot be covered here. However, if you are worried about feeding, do try to get help from your midwife, health visitor, doctor or breastfeeding counsellor.

Chapter Eleven

Working and feeding

'*Several friends and acquaintances, pregnant for the first time, have said wonderingly and hopefully "Oh so it might be possible to breastfeed?", as if this would be a joy which would automatically be denied them as working mothers.*'

More women are combining working outside the home with continuing to offer breastmilk. You may like to investigate options such as job-sharing or part-time work for a while if the baby is very attached to the breast. You may also find that your own – negative – feelings about returning are surprisingly strong: 'The prospect of returning to work loomed ever nearer.'

'*I felt that breastfeeding when I was with them, continued an intimacy and comfort that was very important for all three of us, at a painful time when I was leaving them in a crèche.*'

Your rights

Many people have argued for longer maternity leave so that breastfeeding can be well established before mothers return to work. As legislation changes you will usually find up-to-date details about allowances which are payable and the statutory lengths of maternity leave in the free books given out by maternity units.

There are many variables which can affect a return to work: the age of the baby, the number of feeds still being given and their place in the day, and the hours you are working. It is hard to plan in detail until you see what kind of baby you have and a lot will depend on the childcare you can get. Few workers in our society are able to take the baby with them and feed on demand, but if the baby is in a workplace nursery, or just down the road from the office, there may be no problem about a quick lunchtime breastfeed if the baby is willing. Most mothers, however, find that they are not able to get to their babies during a full day's work.

Some mothers express milk to leave for a childminder or crèche staff to give the baby so that they won't have to use formula; and other mothers use bottled milk when they are not there, and feed the baby themselves when they return home: 'I now bottle feed him (along with his solid food) during the day as I am going back to work . . . but I still breastfeed him last thing at night and this works out very well for us both.' Each mother and baby pair work out their own solutions. This chapter contains several possibilities to start you thinking. An extremely helpful booklet, *Having It All*, is available from the Maternity Alliance (address on page 202). It contains a great deal of useful information about practicalities and your employer's responsibilities towards you as a breastfeeding mother.

Combining bottles and breasts

'We built up from one bottle a week to one a day.'

Introducing a bottle can seem quite important, but it is a good idea to wait a few weeks to make sure the baby is certain of the technique of breastfeeding first. It is difficult to say how much to put in each bottle as the appetite of the baby, and the fat content of each feed, vary so much, and you do not know if the baby will be hungry, or thirsty, or only want comfort and so take a minimum amount and learn to wait for you to return. A very rough guide is to multiply the weight of the baby in pounds by two and a half, and divide by the number of feeds in 24 hours – so a 10-pound baby feeding eight times a day might take around 3 or so ounces a feed. In a bottle or cup your baby may take less than she usually does directly from you; on the other hand, if she is happy to use the alternative method, she may take more. This is because there is likely to be less cream in the milk, as the cream is more difficult to get out by pump. If you are going out for a brief trial period or to a wedding or party it might be an idea to leave several small amounts of milk as it is quite likely that the baby will wait for your return to feed and will take only a little at a time. It would be a great shame to waste a large amount of milk, and when a bottle has been used once it is not a good idea to return to it.

Often babies will take to both bottle and breast with little problem, but do not be surprised if the pattern of the day changes so that night feeds continue for longer than they might otherwise perhaps have done: 'He is six months old now and I still feed him when I get home from work and during the night. I don't really mind the night feeds, it's an opportunity to be close. I don't really wake up much and he comes in and spends the rest of the night in our bed.'

Taking a bottle

When it comes to taking a bottle, some babies are adaptable – some are less so. The following extracts are what some mothers have said about their babies:

- 'The baby would only accept bottles of breastmilk from my husband not from the childminder.'
- 'Initially they refused a bottle from me – for several weeks – but did learn quite quickly (one-two weeks) to take it happily from other people.'
- 'I returned to working for four days a week when Richard was 14 weeks old. He had always been a very accommodating baby, happy to suck anything which was put in his mouth . . . George (second baby) just would not take a bottle from me – or his father – he just knew what he wanted and I think he knew that I didn't really want to give him a bottle.'
- 'we find that if we don't give David a regular bottle (say, once a week) he has to re-learn all about teats and technique.'

Helping your baby to accept a bottle

Try any or all of the following:

- using a cup – a small one for a little baby or a spouted one for a bigger baby may be acceptable to babies who hate bottles
- pouring hot, previously boiled water over the teat to soften and warm it just before you offer it
- someone else offering it
- offering it before the baby is hungry
- giving it after any solids
- tempting the baby with it, so that she takes it, like she does a breast
- offering it in a different position from that used for breastfeeding, eg using a bouncing chair
- facing the baby away from the bottle-giver
- rocking
- using a beaker, spoon or eggcup for milk, holding the baby upright and tilting it gently to offer a sip. Give the baby time to swallow
- if solids are being offered, make them more runny with your milk or with cooled boiled water

Building up stocks

Many women begin to keep frozen breastmilk ready for their return to work: 'I had started expressing after two weeks, just an ounce at first after his feeding had finished. Gradually I built up a stock in the freezer.' If you decide to leave formula for the baby, rather than to express the next day's feed, you will still need to express at work for a while – a little less each day – to reduce

'I've usually fed the baby on one side (sometimes both) and immediately afterwards pumped off whatever milk is left. I've found that the best time of day to do this is first thing in the morning.'

your supply so as to be comfortable, especially if you had been taking off more than the baby needed so as to build up your stocks: 'Every time I reduced a feed I would be in agony with full hard breasts again (for a few days): with expressing regularly you make more milk than you need.'

'I managed to visit the medical centre at work each afternoon, and express milk. (I got quite good at "thinking milk".) I used to pack it in ice, take it home and my son had it the next day.'

Weekends and holidays also raise questions of whether to continue to offer bottles, or to breastfeed entirely. Conflicting support can cause problems with making up your mind: 'The childminder tried to persuade me to bottle-feed every day even though I was only working part-time and the breastfeeding counsellor told me to feed on my days off to keep up the milk supply.'

Finding support

Some NCT branches have working mothers' groups who meet regularly for an evening out – they are also open to pregnant women. If you decide to continue to offer breastmilk, it would be a good idea to think about the possible reactions of colleagues at work to your need to express. It can be quite hard to find supportive friends who understand what you are doing, and difficult to find a place to express your milk in: 'expressing in the school toilets felt quite sordid! But there was nowhere else to go.' It may help to discuss this with your work colleagues before you return.

As usual with breastfeeding, there can be a lot of doubt about a mother's ability to provide satisfactory food for her baby. Working gives fuel for the myth about running out of milk. '. . . others, usually older friends who have not been breastfed . . . are keen to tell me that with Simon to look after and this big old house in the process of being substantially refurbished – by us – I'm bound to be "far too tired to produce proper milk" . . . I'm not impressed.'

Sometimes, the problem is not about milk supply, but about persuading your body to let the milk out for something which is definitely not your own baby! Some women find it helpful to get engrossed in something completely different, especially a conversation.

Your own feelings can affect let-down on a pump as well as for the baby: 'you only have to try pumping after a squabble with your husband or a row with your boss to find out that the best pump in the world won't produce a let-down if you are not in the mood . . . '

Carers

If you normally offer the breast at around the time you get back from work, you may find it helpful to ask your carer to avoid giving a full feed just before. You may need to check that it will be all right for you to sit and feed if the baby is with a carer outside the home.

You may need to warn your carer that human milk can separate , and does not look at all like formula. It is OK as long as it smells all right. It just needs shaking gently.

Expressing milk

Various ways of expressing milk are possible but for many women all forms of expression take quite a lot of getting used to: 'I've stopped feeling embarrassed with close friends or family round me, but I'm not sure I'd want to use a breastpump in a corner of the Ladies at a formal occasion.' Although regular use of a pump, often a battery or mains-driven one, is the most usual and efficient way of getting out large amounts of milk for a baby, you may find it helpful to know how to hand express for other reasons.

Hand expressing

Hand expression takes practice and a good place to do this is in the bath when you have warmth and relaxation on your side, and you don't need to worry at first about trying to catch the milk; you can just practise the technique. Aim to push milk from the reservoirs behind the nipple, and work at getting a let-down so that they keep being refilled just like they are for the baby. These things may help you to get the milk to flow:

- relaxation
- warmth
- stroking the breast all over

Use your fingers and thumb to push back gently into the tissue at the edge of the areola, then squeeze them gently together behind the breast tissue you now have in your hand, rolling a little towards the nipple but not sliding towards it (the baby doesn't). Be careful of bruising yourself, and stop if it hurts. Move around the areola edge, and switch sides when you get tired or if the milk is coming more slowly – it is quite usual to have drips at first.

Hand-held breast pumps

There are many kinds of hand pumps, some working like bicycle pumps with inner and outer cylinders which slide up and down, or towards and away from you, and some with trigger handles so that you can operate them one-handed. If friends will let you see how they work this gives you a good idea about what might suit you. The little glass and rubber 'breast relievers' which look like old-fashioned car horns and are available on prescription, are not actually true breast pumps at all as it is not possible to sterilise them.

Electric pumps

Small electric pumps, some using mains electricity, and some using batteries (rechargable ones save on a lot of replacement batteries), are also available. Some mothers like the ones on which you use your own thumb to control the rate of suction as the rate of expression can then be varied in response to the flow of your milk. Large electric breast pumps work very efficiently but are heavy. Some like their action – 'the gentle rhythmic hum

---

'Ages of pumping gave very little milk, but I persevered. Eventually I was able to get out a fair amount (6–8oz).'

Making expressing easier

- feeding the baby and pumping at the same time
- expressing when you feel very full – the baby can still get more out
- expressing if you have a spontaneous let-down
- making yourself comfortable, perhaps in the same place each time so as to get your body used to letting milk down for the baby
- having a photograph of the baby or something she has worn nearby as you 'feed' the pump
- relaxing – it is easy to say to someone you have to be calm to allow let-down so you can express into a pump. Remember that every drop helps, and if you are upset or frustrated, acknowledge this at least to yourself. It may well help to speak to someone.
- massaging your breasts before or after during expression
- hand expressing, which helps hormonally and gives more hindmilk
- massaging the 'other' breast and nipple while you express may help
- getting someone to rub your back between the shoulder blades and backbone with their fists (one going up while the other goes down). This works best if you have no clothes between you, but you helper needs to use oil to prevent rubbing on your skin
- expressing after you have fed the baby (if you are breast-feeding sometimes) – there will be useful hormones still circulating in your body (though you may not expect as much milk)
- an attachment available from one or two firms allows both breasts to be expressed at once, saving time and possibly raising hormone levels usefully
- there is also an inner ridged soft plastic liner which seems to help

of the machine relaxed me and I could feel the let-down reflex' –
others do not.

A breastfeeding counsellor will be able to give you up-to-date
information about what is currently available and discuss what
you feel might be the best thing for you.

Storing breast milk

Milk needs to be cooled down quickly, kept in the main part of
the fridge and either frozen within a day or used within a day or
so. Everything used should be sterile, or in the case of your
hands, as clean as possible. It should keep for a couple of weeks
in a little in-fridge freezer and for at least three months in a
proper freezer. Milk can be thawed at room temperature or in a
container of hot water. Microwaving is not recommended. You
may notice the milk separating into two layers as you thaw it.
Nothing is wrong; it is just the fat floating to the top. Shaking
will mix it.

You will also need freezing bags or good quality plastic con-
tainers to freeze the milk in, an insulated cool bag, and ice-packs
from a chemist or camping shop for taking milk home if you
have expressed at work, or from home to the baby's carer. It is
safer to prevent cling film containing PVC from touching the
milk. Some mothers use a sterilised ice tray to freeze their milk
and then store the cubes in a plastic tub or bag. You can get special bags for saving breast milk.

A breastfeeding counsellor may be able to help with suggestions at a practical level and also, if you wish, take time to listen
as you prepare to combine working and feeding or if you find
you have mixed feelings about what you are doing. Some of the
points about expressing milk on page 159 may also help.

CHAPTER TWELVE

Special mothers and babies

'I breastfed both of my children although it was difficult with my first as he has a genetic disorder. He was very slow at sucking and each feed took well over an hour.'

All babies are special for their parents, and many go through crises or problems, but some are 'special' for a long time, or for life. There are implications in several problems in babies and mothers for breastfeeding. Your own shock at having had a baby who is not fully well can make thinking about the practicalities of breastfeeding seem an added difficulty in itself, but you can, with help, hope at least for some breastfeeding for many special babies. For all special babies, breastmilk is an obvious precious source of protection against infection, and many mothers therefore want to begin breastfeeding, and see how things go. Expressing milk with a pump, especially to get to calorie-rich hindmilk, may help some babies who cannot feed for long or very effectively.

Feeding may be more time-consuming for many babies, such as those with heart problems who tire easily, or those with neurological damage who do not easily learn to suck, swallow and breathe in a very coordinated way at first.

Supporting such babies all along their bodies may help to keep them feeding longer, and avoiding a lying-down position which encourages sleep. Changing sides so that the baby is stimulated – and so are lots of little let-downs in you – or expressing some milk from behind the areola into the baby's mouth may encourage her. To hold the jaw and breast stable together, an American idea is to cup your hand under your breast with your thumb and finger on either side of the areola, and slide the thumb and index finger forward to support the baby, gently resting them against the baby's cheeks. Babies with Down's syndrome may be rather floppy and not feed very well at first. It has been found helpful to stimulate the tongue with little sucking movements before feeding.

Whole books have been written about mothers and babies with all kinds of special needs, and if your particular situation is not covered in this short section, do try the health professions and your breastfeeding support organisations to see if there are ways around the difficulties. Your surgeon, or doctor may not have met a situation where a mother wishes to continue to breastfeed before. However, support groups may well have accounts of women who have managed to continue feeding or to resume feeding despite interruptions and traumas. Likewise, a breastfeeding counsellor can get hold of a special situations register holder to try to put you in touch with other parents who have had a similar concern. This does not mean that they will be able to solve everything, or contradict what the health professionals have told you, but they may be one step further along the road and be able to help you think about strategies for practical ways around problems, as well as understanding your feelings more readily.

Premature babies

It can be a great sadness and shock to find that your pregnancy ends before you were expecting it to. You may not yet have attended enough antenatal classes to feel physically or emotionally prepared for labour. You will find that your baby and you are separated and that perhaps the baby is not well. When you are able to see your baby, she will look unlike the others on the ward who are with their mothers, because she will be smaller and less chubby and be in a special incubator with monitors and tubes taped into place.

'My daughter was premature – 29 weeks and 2½lbs, and was in special care for eight weeks.'

If you were hoping that there would be little medical intervention in the birth, you are suddenly in a world which is unfamiliar. There are strange noises and lights in a Special Care Baby Unit or Neonatal Intensive Care Unit (SCBU or NICU for short). Tiny babies sleep for long periods as they would have done in the womb and they need to be woken regularly for feeds. Test weighing may still be used to ensure that the baby is getting what is needed. As medical advances have been made, improving the outcome for very tiny babies, the SCBU staff have also become more aware of the need for parents to be involved in the care of their babies. Some babies, for example, go home still on oxygen therapy.

You and your partner will soon be able to build up a relationship with the staff and ask for explanations about worries you may have. For them, as for you, the priority is to keep the baby well while she catches up, and help her to grow so that she can go home, but long-term breastfeeding may be higher on the agenda for you, so it is worth explaining what you hope for. For example, it may be possible to ask for the baby to be tube-fed and later cup-fed if necessary, rather than bottle-fed, as steps towards breastfeeding. You may sometimes be able to offer your own milk by tube when this begins.

If you are able to, it may help to put in your hand and stroke her gently to begin to let her know that you are there. Progress can often be rapid after the baby gets used to having been born early, but setbacks are also common as tiny babies are very prone to other problems, such as infections and jaundice.
In these circumstances, it is hard to start thinking about the practicalities of breastfeeding a baby who is perhaps weeks away from even trying to suckle at the breast, and it can feel like a big risk to begin this process which means you are hoping that all will eventually be well.

Starting to express milk right away will encourage your milk supply and means you will be able to freeze colostrum ready to give to your baby as soon as she is able to take food by tube.

Hand expressing can be particularly helpful in getting the naturally small amounts of colostrum and milk available for your baby at this time and awakening your breasts to action. Very small babies may be fed directly into the vein, and will move then to tube feeding into the stomach or intestine when they can begin to digest expressed milk. Only tiny amounts will be needed, around a teaspoonful an hour, and every drop is useful to the baby, especially for preventing infection, and for brain growth. If you use the pump in the hospital it is a good idea to try it on a gentle setting at first, working up to the point where suction is stronger but comfortable.

It means too, that your breasts will begin to respond by changing to making milk. This is different from the milk of full-term baby's mothers, with more of the things that premature babies need, particularly protein and some minerals. After a while it becomes the same as other mothers' milk. This means that some babies who are going to be a long time in the SCBU will need extra formula as well. One expert suggests asking to have your own milk mixed with any formula felt to be necessary so that enzymes helping digestion can be present all the time. Fat from your milk sticks to the tubes and will usually be washed out with a little water so that the baby gets every drop of goodness. Currently there are 13 milk banks in hospitals, where pooled and pasteurised milk donated by breastfeeding mothers is available for premature babies. The number of milk banks is slowly rising as the value of human milk for these very special babies is better appreciated.

'When I look back I feel so pleased that we managed it in the end, as I feel it helped him get over his poor start.'

While you are in the hospital it should be possible to use an electric breast pump to express milk for your baby. It may be kept in the unit which is busy, but near the baby, helping you to let milk down. When you go home, the hospital may be able to let you have one or you may need to hire one. Electric pumps can

> *'I found it difficult to feel anything for him. I had no
> desire to stay with him in hospital . . . however I was
> keen to breastfeed from both the convenience point of
> view and from the knowledge that breastmilk really
> would be best for Stephen.'*

be hired from the NCT and other agents in most areas of the country. Ask your maternity hospital or the NCT. The agents will be able to help you with information. They are sometimes breastfeeding counsellors, or they will always be able to put you in touch with one.

Mothers do not find it easy to use a breast pump several times a day and yet this is vital to keep your milk supply going for the baby. There are some guidelines at the end of this chapter. 'I hired an electric breast pump which I used every three hours. Initially the babies were fed with formula and a little of my colostrum. After a few days I was able to provide half their feeds and then all of them. That was a big thing for me. I felt so estranged from them since I couldn't put them to the breast, but at least they were receiving my milk through the tube. I was taught to manage the whole operation, but would not have coped at all well emotionally, had it not been for another wonderful community midwife, who in fact was based with the special care unit. She talked me through, helping me to plan a strict timetable, to keep the milk stimulated. I started pumping at 6am then at 9am, then 12.00, so that I could be at the hospital for their 12.30 feed . . . '

Going home without the baby

At home you may feel very lonely without your partner if he has returned to work, wondering about your baby left behind in hospital. You might be able to leave a breastpad with your milk on it behind in the crib so that the baby can remember you while you are away. If you have another child, visiting the new baby can be difficult without extended support.

A lot of your time will be taken up with expressing milk and washing or sterilising the pump accessories and visiting the baby.

The hospital will probably give you guidelines for pumping and storing milk.

Coming out of the incubator

Each stage may be longed for and yet lead to some fearfulness for you. Guidance from medical staff is obviously paramount in this, over whether the baby is ready to be outside the safe environment of the incubator, whether she can maintain her temperature alone, and later coordinate suckling, swallowing and breathing. Until this is tested it is difficult to know. Many babies' reactions used to be tested by first feeding them by bottle, but more hospitals are now feeling that time with the baby held against you, getting to know how you feel and smell will help her to breastfeed later, and may help to encourage your milk. Holding the baby in your arms for the first time will be possible, and this is another stage towards being able to feed her directly: 'the midwife taught me to tube feed the babies next to my breasts, then gradually allow sucking at the same time, until their reflex was strong enough.'

'. . . the real need for mothers with babies on special care is to get enough rest. I was encouraged to spend a lot of time there . . . special care units are not very relaxing places. I was just totally exhausted by the time she came home.'

There is no need to rush into trying out breastfeeding. Mouthing and licking, like a newborn baby, is more likely at first, and then it will be up to you to watch for her to make a move: 'At about 31 weeks gestation I noticed my baby rooting and then on I put her to my breast at every visit: at least twice a day. By 34 weeks gestation she was sucking very well, although it tired her and she still needed to be fed (my milk) by naso-gastric tube. By 35 weeks gestation she was taking alternate feeds from me or from a bottle of expressed milk.'

The stage between the baby being allowed out for holding and full breastfeeding may be quite a long period, and even when breastfeeding begins, initially it is likely only to be allowed once or twice a day. It is quite a balancing act between feeding the baby and exhausting her by trying. After around 30 weeks or more and weighing around 1500 gams, a baby may begin to try to breastfeed if she is well. If the baby is needing extra oxygen, this can be blown across her face by someone else while you feed for a short time each day, before she is topped up with a tube or bottle-fed.*

Some hospitals now agree that breastfeeding is less work than bottle-feeding for the premature baby, as the mother is, after all, squeezing down the milk and a premature baby finds it easier to suck and swallow together in breastfeeding than in bottle-feeding.

First feeds

It can be difficult to feed in a SCBU. Ideally, you need pillows, privacy, and a supportive member of staff to help. Midwives are there to support your breastfeeding so ask for their experienced help if you are feeling in need of it. 'He had shown no interest at all previously. With the midwife's help, and quite a lot of patience, I managed to introduce him to the breast eventually. It was hard work, as the chairs were not at all comfortable, the room was 84 degrees and there was no privacy.'

It may help to look at how to position babies at the breast on pages 25–34. Many things will be the same, but some are different. Premature babies tend to curl up and you need to support their whole body. Using a pillow, or the underarm hold may help. You may need to support the baby's head gently while she feeds.

Massaging your breast and stimulating your nipple to make it ready for her as well as expressing a little milk first may help to encourage her, but do not worry if you cannot see milk, it is there for the baby. As tiny babies tire quickly, it may be a good idea to let the baby feed on one breast rather than split the feed into two short ones. She can then reach the hindmilk.

The baby may not always be ready to feed well, and it may help to know that a study has shown that any sucking, even on dummies (which may teach babies unhelpful mouth movements), can help premature babies to digest milk given by tube. This means that even periods of not very effective suckling may be very useful, not only in reminding your breasts to make more milk for the baby, but in helping the baby to make the most of what she receives by the tube.

It is a good idea to say when you are coming to the hospital and then try to stick to the time, so that a bottle- or tube-feed is not given if you are hoping to breastfeed. 'Once or twice I felt very angry when I was five minutes late and the staff had gone ahead and fed them formula. I made big notices for their cots.'

Feeding a premature baby can need a lot of patience as the baby may take a while to rouse, and may need to lick and smell you first for a while. The staff will need to know how feeds are going in terms of time and the expected schedules may be difficult to follow for everyone.

Coming home

Prior to coming home, there are usually a few rooms available at the hospital for mothers to get the feel of a whole day and night with their babies. 'At 36 weeks I went to stay in the hospital again for two nights and did all her feeds.' Again, though, a longed-for stage can sometimes make a mother feel a bit uncertain. 'I was desperate to take them home and yet worried that they weren't getting enough.'

Policies about discharge vary with the hospital; perhaps they will look at the weight of the baby, or assess the babies' development individually. Once home, the support of other mothers can be kept up and the hospital usually has some kind of liaison professional, and you can always ring back to the Unit if you are worried.

You may well still be giving complementary feeds when you go home but hoping to cut these down slowly as your milk supply increases with the stimulation of your own baby. 'The hard work continued when we came home, as I had to increase my supply for him. The end result was that I fed him myself until he was seven months old, when both he and I decided mutually to stop.'

When the baby comes home, you may feel recovered from the birth even if you had a caesarean but it is still a tremendous responsibility and hard work to care for a baby for the first time, and especially one who has been in special care. Just explaining to everyone why she is so small and how old you feel she *really* is can be hard work. This is a new time to accept any offers of help – like someone doing the ironing or making you a cake or casserole. Time is what you are being offered and it is the most precious gift, since it frees you to sleep or eat or spend time with the baby or your partner without feeling so exhausted.

You may need to wake the baby for regular feeds if she is still sleepy, but later she may be fretful and need breastfeeding a great deal as a comfort after the hard time she has had. It is a good idea to try to feed roughly two to three hourly during the day, with a longer sleep at night. Keeping the pump for a couple of weeks to build up milk supply and perhaps offering expressed hindmilk by spoon or small cup if the baby is not able to feed for very long at a time can help her growth to be as good as possible.

Expressing milk for ill or premature babies

If your baby is unable to breastfeed, for whatever reason, and you wish to feed her purely with breastmilk, these things may help you to use an electric pump more efficiently:

- moistening the breast to get a good suction
- making sure your nipple is central in the funnel
- not pressing the funnel hard into your breast or you stop the milk flowing and could cause pressure on ducts.
- short frequent feeds often work better than a few longer ones
- working up to expressing for five minutes a side or longer for up to eight times a day, returning to each breast in turn until the milk is no longer flowing
- hand expressing after the pump has got as much milk as it can and to stimulate let-down
- trying first thing in the morning and very last thing at night, like a baby would
- trying night feeds, eg if you get up anyway it could be worth even expressing a little by hand to encourage the flow, even if you did not save the milk
- see also pages 156–159

Because the baby's store of iron was not complete when born, she has to be given supplements such as vitamins and iron syrups in addition to breastmilk which is by now catering for a term baby. If you are worried that the baby is keener on a bottle than on feeding from you, you can use a spoon.

Cleft lips and palates

One of the more common difficulties for breastfeeding is a range of problems with babies' mouths including cleft lips and palates. Each cleft lip is in a different place, and, while waiting for treatment, some babies may be able to feed in particular positions on the breast if the breast tissue – or a well-placed finger – is able to fill up the gap. One breast may fit better than the other and it is worth trying an underarm hold or one where the baby faces you fairly upright on your lap. Cleft lips can be operated on at any time between a few days and three months. You will probably be shown photographs of babies who have also had operations which give you hope about the future. Different surgeons have varying approaches about the length of time after the operation which must pass before breastfeeding can begin again.

A hole in the palate means a baby cannot properly create enough suction to hold on to the breast, and air can get in easily through the nose, meaning the baby may have a lot of wind and often will need extra time to bring it up. Also, milk may come down her nose, harmlessly. Feeding the baby in a semi-upright position may help to lessen this. Lying down while supporting the baby's head may also make feeding possible, and an orthodontic plate may be made to cover the hole – being shaped anew as the baby grows. You will be given guidance about other ways of feeding babies who cannot use an ordinary teat or the breast for the time being; special teats and spoon attachments on bottles have been developed. A repair to the hard palate may be done at about six months onwards and at six or eight years for the soft palate. There is helpful information in a pamphlet from the Cleft Lip and Palate Association (see page 199). If your baby has a cleft lip, you are likely to find yourself maintaining breastmilk on a pump, so it may help to look at page 169.

Hip disorders

Babies with 'clicky' hips, or congenital hip disorders, can have a lot more done now so that they will be straight and well as adults. In the short term, however, some of the procedures can affect breastfeeding. In some cases, the baby will need to go into hospital for traction for some weeks. Mothers who have experienced this have found it possible to maintain breastfeeding by leaning over the cot and dangling their breast into the baby's mouth. Babies are surprisingly adaptable, and if they are hungry, this rather strange way of feeding will seem fine to them. If the baby has to be in a 'broomstick plaster' to keep her legs even further apart, the plaster will have to be changed under a general anaesthetic every two or three months, or in the case of a younger child even more often. (Chapter 10 may help you begin to think about hospitalisation.)

Mothers with extra challenges

It is unusual for breasts to be badly injured even though they do seem quite vulnerable. After a car accident, for example, the seat belts may have damaged the duct system and blood may come out for a while with the milk, but this will not harm the baby. Scalds and burns from accidents before pregnancy may not affect milk production, as much of the work of cell-making happens then. Damage to the nipple itself might mean it would be difficult for milk to be transferred to the baby, but each situation will be different, with scarred skin taking time to regain elasticity, and you may want to speak to your midwife or doctor and ask to be referred to a specialist.

Operations for breast increase, where a silicone bag has been inserted between the chest wall and breast tissue, are not supposed to interfere with milk production. The bags may be felt, however, as the breasts begin to grow during pregnancy and work during lactation. Breast reductions, where the milk ducts may have been cut, may lead to some difficulties. But the ducts sometimes rejoin themselves depending on whether the nipple was resited, and how long ago it is since the operation. It may be possible to speak to the surgeon who did the operation. If you still have a sense of feeling in your nipple and surrounding skin then this is very helpful for milk production. Surgery for cysts and tumours may affect the production or delivery of milk, but nevertheless you may feel it is worth trying to breastfeed, remembering that it is perfectly possible to feed a baby via one breast alone. If you have had a lumpectomy, your surgeon will have thoughts on whether it is a good idea to breastfeed or not, depending on how long it is since your operation.

If you have to have surgery during breastfeeding you will need to discuss with your surgeon whether it is advisable for you to continue to breastfeed after the operation. It is not necessary to interrupt breastfeeding for a mammograph in which the breast is X-rayed. If you are unfortunate enough to be found to have a malignant lump, all treatments for cancer after operations mean that breastfeeding must stop for the sake of the baby. Women who have had mastectomies and subsequent clean bills of health have gone on to feed their babies from the remaining breast alone.

Postnatal depression

This affects a lot of mothers mildly, and a very few severely. Some mothers feel breastfeeding is an extra burden during this debilitating period, while others find it is one thing they enjoy and feel they can do well.

'I did not feel that my mothering skills were too good but my growing baby enabled me to see that I had got at least one aspect of motherhood right.'

It may take some time for you, or others, to realise quite how bad you are feeling. One mother (above, right) who wrote her account of breastfeeding for this book found it gave her the opportunity to look back at her experience.

When discussing drug therapy with your doctor the question of continuing to breastfeed may come up. If you feel you are not likely to be able to put your point of view across sufficiently well, you might like to ask your partner or a friend who knows how

'I realised that I'd had a lousy year and that it probably wasn't normal to feel this angry and anxious about the baby. I went to my doctor and my health visitor: was diagnosed as suffering from postnatal depression and have just begun a course of psychotherapy and anti-depressants.

'Fortunately, my doctor was very supportive. He prescribed anti-depressants which I was reluctant to try until he assured me that these ones would not harm Alice. As the anti-depressants worked, I became more relaxed and my milk supply improved.'

you feel about continuing to breastfeed to go with you because, 'depression . . . is not a condition that puts one in a frame of mind to "tackle" anyone with a high probability of success.'

HIV and AIDS

It was first realised in 1985 that it was possible to transmit the HIV virus to babies through breastmilk, and later that a baby who was infected might give it to her mother. Currently, the Department of Health has said that mothers in high risk groups and those who are already HIV-positive should not breastfeed. A talk to your doctor about this may help if you feel this may apply to you. Research is being undertaken into this aspect of AIDs, as it is towards finding a vaccine and cures.

Diabetic mothers

Your specialist and dietician are obviously going to offer impor-tant guidance, as your insulin level will need to be adjusted, just as it was in pregnancy. But after the first few days of carefully watching the baby and you, breastfeeding can work very well. It is, in fact, a gentle way to make the transition to the pre-preg-nant state, because insulin requirements are lower on the whole than normal. The baby may be more likely to have low blood sugar and jaundice, both of which can make the beginnings of breastfeeding harder, so it may help to look at the sections dealing with those problems (see pages 57 and 59). Your milk may come in slightly later than other mothers' too, but it is particularly worth persevering despite any initial problems, since research has shown that managing without formula can help protect a baby whose parent has insulin-dependent diabetes from developing the same condition. Slow weaning is especially important for mothers with diabetes.

Wheelchair users

You may well have been expected to have a caesarean, and so begin with even more difficulties, but wheelchair users who responded to our request for information found nurses very helpful with establishing breastfeeding.

If the disability or other symptoms such as arthritis are quite enough to make life with a baby difficult, but not sufficiently severe to mean you get a lot of help, you may have to be especially inventive and patient about such areas as positioning the baby. Some mothers experience painful wrists during pregnancy and lactation, caused by retained fluid trapping a nerve. Your health visitor may be able to arrange some home help for you.

'While I was pregnant, my GP checked up on the drugs I was taking to see if there was any chance they would go into breast milk. Luckily, my MS improved so much that I stopped taking them after about the fourth month of pregnancy. When my daughter was about 11 months old the beneficial effects of pregnancy had just about disappeared, so I stopped breastfeeding and started the tablets again.'

Chronic illness

Fatigue and drugs may present problems so it is worth remembering that breastfeeding can be a restful period. Drugs are, of course, a medical matter but letting doctors know if breastfeeding is a priority for you, may override an assumption that it will be too tiring or incompatible with treatment.

Relactation

This may be a choice after an interruption to breastfeeding following an illness and drug treatment, the realisation that a baby has an allergy to formula, or changing your mind about bottles. It is also a term sometimes used when breastfeeding is begun when a mother is going to feed a baby she has not given birth to herself. After a gap in feeding, it is often possible to return to full or partial breastfeeding simply by putting the baby to the breast, offering fewer and fewer, and smaller and smaller complementary feeds – if she will cooperate – and building up the milk supply while watching her nappies and weight gain. (See page 139 for more information about weaning a baby off bottles.)

Feeding an adopted baby

If you are considering feeding an adopted baby you will be beginning from scratch, even if you have fed a baby before. If you have never been pregnant, it may well be more difficult for you to make a full supply of milk. While the chance of making a total milk supply for a baby is not certain, the chance of getting some milk is good. It is worth talking to others to find out about what is involved in breastfeeding. You may be interested to hear how far the breast is seen as a comforter as well as a source of food. Think about what you are actually hoping for – a full milk supply, to feel like a 'real mother', to be able sometimes to offer what one mother called 'a special cuddle', or to be able to keep the baby happy on the breast when you warm a bottle. You will need to discuss your aims with your partner and the agency workers who may well be supportive.

If you are getting a young baby this will obviously make it more likely that she will be willing to suckle at the breast, but for a few days while she settles it may be helpful to offer her the bottle at times she may have been used to it. To help her in general to increase her awareness of you as her new care-giver, put a piece of clothing you have worn in the cot next to her.

It can help to begin to express some milk gradually before the baby arrives – if you know when this is. Begin slowly and carefully and don't panic if little comes for some time: the baby is a lot better at making the system work. It can be useful to continue

Some encouraging moves for relactation

The following ideas have all been tried:

- offering the breast first, and/or after the bottle
- expressing a little milk first to get it flowing
- using a nursing supplementer (see page 176)
- feeding in the same place each time
- feeding in a dim light, with music, rocking, etc
- skin to skin contact
- relaxation for you and massage for the baby
- offering a night feed (at this time hormone levels are high)
- avoiding heavy perfumes and letting the baby get used to you
- feeding in the bath
- feeding the baby half-asleep
- changing to an 'orthodontic' teat which may be less unlike a nipple
- using a teat with a smaller hole
- mixing expressed breast milk with the baby's formula

using a pump for extra stimulation once the baby has taught your body what is needed. (For help with using breast-pumps, see pages 156 and 169.)

Some mothers have found it helpful to use a 'supplementer' – a bag or bottle of expressed or formula milk with a tube attached which is taped on to the mother's areola and so allows the baby to have some encouraging milk while she suckles to build up a supply.

After a week or so, assess how things are going. It is worth asking whether you and the baby are enjoying what is happening, as well as if there is beginning to be milk. Do seek support in this venture if you can before you begin, as you may be able to start 'priming' your body to feed a baby before she arrives by using certain drugs (see information about the National Childbirth Trust, page 192).

CHAPTER THIRTEEN

Stopping

'I have gone through a great deal of soul-searching. Why was I doing it? Who was it for? What would be for the best?'

It can seem unbelievable that within a week a baby who has fed for every day of her life may have forgotten how to do it, or that a baby who has made breastfeeding such an important part of her life will one day show signs of greater interest in other sources of food and comfort. Not only may you feel that your baby needs to be weaned from your milk and from you, but you may also feel for many reasons that you need to wean yourself from this important part of your relationship. An increasing minority of women are quietly feeding their babies well into the second and third years. If you embark on this worthwhile option you may well feel you could do with finding support in this easy way of comforting and feeding a toddler. Society in general is, to say the least, surprised to see a baby with teeth, speech, shoes or any other signs of independence returning to his mother for breastfeeds in between playing with others or after a tumble. Try contacting your local breastfeeding support organisation to be put in touch with other members. Many women and those around them feel it can be difficult letting the baby decide when to wean herself because it can be so unpredictable. Once the baby is older than about a year, it can become more of a problem for the mother to stop breastfeeding against the baby's wishes.

Initially, as you continue happily to breastfeed people will leave you alone with your decision, but as their idea of the time for weaning approaches, they may begin to become very interested again. 'Oliver is now ten months old . . . I sense equal measures of disapproval and wonder at the fact that I am still breastfeeding him and am not attempting to stop.' They may have a genuine concern for you, the baby, or your marriage, and wonder about another baby. Other ideas come into play, about controlling babies – about spoiling and over-dependence – and babies beginning to 'enjoy' breastfeeding in a way which others may find hard to cope with. In all this, it is helpful to be making decisions as a partnership if you are in one. You can seek support for deciding, or for continuing breastfeeding from a breastfeeding organisation.

'I decided to give her a bottle in the evenings, as she'd always been a "sucky" baby, but had never sucked her thumb, and it seemed a bit hard suddenly to deprive her of her comfort habit.'

If you do decide to stop feeding, from the baby's point of view, the kinds of questions you need to ask yourself about not offering the breast are about what kind of substitutes to offer. These not only concern the milk 'container', and whether she might still enjoy a bottle or be an independent soul who already likes her own beaker, but all the other things which a feed gives her. Unboiled doorstep milk is not recommended as a drink until the baby is a year old; goat's milk is not recommended because of an increased disease risk. Also, according to the Royal College of Midwives, there is no advantage in the follow-on milks over ordinary formula.

An older baby may be finding feeding very consoling at times of stress for her – teething, illnesses, moving house, having visitors, beginning at a new nursery: 'we would be moving across the country. This couldn't be the right time to wean.' Cuddles and rocking will replace suckling now. Some alternative rituals for bedtime, and for daytime sleeps may be necessary when the cosy warmth of a breastfeed is gone. Apart from stories, these might include cuddles, stroking, baths, time with fathers, and grandparents. Some things may help – soft toys, the satin edges of blankets, or muslin nappies – or try putting your tee-shirt in the cot with the baby. The baby is losing food, drink, sucking, intimate contact, time with you and immediate comfort: it can take care to replace these aspects of her life. A story read on your knee while she strokes or holds to her face your hair, a favourite cloth or a teddy may help to make the transition. Sometimes, especially perhaps if she has had her needs met, you may find the baby surprisingly casual: 'The last feed was very sad for me, but I don't think Jonathan even noticed.'

Many mothers find their older babies feed partly out of boredom, or when they see you sitting down, so you may have to avoid this for a few days. It may help to distract the baby by being out all day with other mothers, and children who are not still feeding.

Night feeds

These seem particularly to figure in parents' thinking about giving up breastfeeding. If they are still frequent, you may feel that stopping breastfeeding altogether may well give the baby less incentive for staying awake when she stirs. If these are the last feeds to go, it can be quite hard to stop them – there is little distraction to offer in the night – and you may feel an older baby's cries sound very loud to neighbours in the early hours.

It is certainly worth discussing this problem with your partner, if this is possible. Finding some time to talk together about your feelings is a priority, although the very situation can make it hard to find time to talk now about, for example, whether your partner feels pushed out by the baby being in bed. If you are wishing to conceive again and finding you lack the opportunity, or that feeding is so frequent that the contraceptive effect is still stopping ovulation, you obviously need to talk with each other.

A weekend or holiday provides a time when perhaps a partner might go to the baby with alternatives ranging from bananas, drinks of water, rocking and singing or staying with her. Other possibilities are often suggested in books about sleep and basically boil down to leaving the baby for very short, perhaps increasing, times to cry, then offering reassurance and settling in the cot, until she gives up. With a mobile child, you may have to sleep firmly on your stomach for a while. Managing to stop breastfeeding is not a guarantee of the end of night waking, of course.

You

From your point of view, gradual weaning is to be preferred if you have a choice. You might cut out alternate feeds, from the middle of the baby's day, one by one, ideally taking a week or two over each one at least, and gradually working towards giving one late or early feed for several weeks so that you do not get uncomfortable. You will probably end up with whichever feed you both enjoy most – either an early one in bed, or a late one when you feel relaxed.

---

*'She has a feed every ten days or two weeks . . .
each one may always be the last – and is very
precious to me.'*

Whenever you stop breastfeeding suddenly, you may be physically as well as emotionally distressed. Milk stays in the breast, and sometimes leaks for several months, as it is gradually reabsorbed by the body. It is easy to underestimate the amount being given in a few short feeds and a long bedtime or early morning suck, especially if some feeds are given at night while you are half asleep. Engorgement can be painful. Keeping your breasts lump-free by gentle massage, and expressing the minimum milk while wearing a supporting bra which does not cut into you will help. Cabbage leaves inside the bra will help too, as will cold compresses, and leaking into the bath.

When circumstances decide

If you feel that the end of breastfeeding is being forced upon you it can be very difficult to accept.

Chapter 9 on Overcoming crises may help you, or you may find there is a way round your situation. Some mothers wrote of the most dismal scenarios from which they were rescued by expert help at the right time.

One such mother tells of her copious milk supply, but that her baby had never learned the proper act of positioning and suckling: 'The baby was now nine days old and feeding him was taking all my time. By the end of the week my mother had to go back to work and I was still having to use the nipple shield, pump and top-ups . . . I cried. I made up the bottles. It seemed only practical . . . next day I mourned for my milk.

'. . . I gave two further feeds when I was engorged – the only way Henry was getting enough milk from me was by let-down reflex, not sucking. It has taken me a long time to realise that that was the problem. He wasn't getting enough in his mouth to suck and stimulate the process properly . . . I still partly blamed myself although they said it was the baby's fault.

'We went on a week's family holiday and on our return my longing for breastfeeding got worse . . . I thought about relactation . . . after one-and-a-half weeks I found I could now make almost half of his milk.

'Nine weeks old. A breakthrough. A midwife friend puts me in touch with an experienced midwife . . . after a token fight from Henry he was latched on and feeding . . . the next day I didn't have to give any formula till 2pm. The next day it was 6.30pm.' When fully breastfeeding, this proud mother wrote: 'This is indeed the greatest achievement of my life.'

The sad truth is, though, that there may not be enough skilled help around when breastfeeding is going really badly, with pain for the mother or failure to thrive in the baby. Or the situation may be beyond assistance or simply beyond your

---

'It hurt, it hurt a lot more than anyone will ever know.'

'At the time I felt it was the worst thing that had ever happened to me . . . '

'Though I loved and still do love him passionately I got out of giving him the hated bottles whenever I could . . .'

---

endurance: 'I felt such relief when I decided to give up and bottle-feed.'

But you may be left with a new problem.

Feelings

For just a few women, the decision to stop will be absolutely forced upon them, by drug treatment in illness or other traumatic events, but usually the decision is less definite. There can be a feeling of 'if only I'd tried harder' about it, or that the decision was not entirely yours. This is one reason why, if you are able to choose, it is a good idea to wait until a crisis – the third bout of mastitis, for example – has passed, before making your decision to stop or to go on trying. Later you will then know you had time to think about things without the extra pressure of feeling grim. This may be the first big thing you tried, and feel you failed in, or it may be the first time your body did not quite do what you wanted. *You* cannot fail in bottle-feeding because it is not entirely your responsibility, but breastfeeding does have this risk, so in deciding to do it in the first place, you have already offered your baby something very special, a gift of hope in yourself.

Not having expected difficulties – seeing breastfeeding as a natural process which everyone can do – can lead to feelings of inadequacy in your mothering abilities, especially in comparison with others.

'I didn't want to be seen struggling at something I thought should have come naturally', and:

'. . . my three closest friends who all delivered within a month of me were all happily breastfeeding without any problems at all.'

Coming to terms with stopping

You are happy to have stopped, or if you regret it but feel you are coming to terms with that, that is fine. 'My husband found me in tears and suggested switching to bottle-feeding. This I did, and it was the best decision I could have made – at that time.' But it is not always like that: 'Now that my milk could be seen in bottles . . . comparatively "thin and white", the "quality" was being questioned. It felt as though every close family member was pressuring me to give up and by the time he was five months, I had totally given up feeding him. I always regretted that and when I had my second child, despite the same lack of family support, I breastfed her until almost a year, which felt right for both me and her.'

'There is also part of me, that to my surprise, is glad she is no longer breastfeeding. Until she was weaned from me, I hadn't been aware of how often I resented her demands for feeding, especially in the morning when I felt at my worst, and just wanted to sleep.'

'All I had known was pain, boredom, resentment and desperation.'

'After I had decided to give up attempting to breastfeed I spent about two hours in a hot bath,, staring down at my useless breasts, sobbing and saying "I tried, I did try, I did," over and over again.'

'I have learnt to be much more flexible in my approach and not to be too hard on myself.'

Individual reactions to any experience felt as 'failure' can vary tremendously, including never wanting to have anything to do with the whole business again, blaming those who could have helped more, or deciding to be assertive in asking for help next time. 'This time I decided to ask for help from anyone who could . . . as I had had virtually no help from midwifery staff when trying to feed Ellie, and I had been too "shy" to ask.'

Talking can help

Others cannot know exactly what you have been through on your way to your decision or understand your need to mourn what you may feel you have lost: 'some had the attitude that I "just didn't try hard enough".'

If you find you are going over and over the circumstances in your head, and not getting a satisfactory resolution, or if seeing another woman breastfeeding makes you very upset, do give yourself time to talk about your feelings to someone who understands so that you can try to come to terms with what has happened.

'I wish I'd known more about the NCT in those days . . . a valuable contact for talking to other mums many of whom had also had problems with breastfeeding. It helped me feel less of a failure.'

'I telephoned (the breastfeeding counsellor) and arranged a visit so that I could cry on her shoulder. We spent many hours going over what had happened and more importantly over my feelings, so that I could come to terms with my "failure". These sessions were of tremendous importance to me.'

However abruptly, carefully or sadly a baby stops feeding, there is some regret involved, for the end of breastfeeding is the beginning of the end of a very special part of babyhood, and the tentative beginning of a new journey towards independence in a child who will ultimately be quite separate from us.

CHAPTER FOURTEEN

Passing it on

'I am in debt to all the people who listened and who shared their own experience with me. With their support and the help of the breastfeeding counsellors I was able to make an informed choice as to whether I would persevere or not. If I had decided to bottle-feed the baby, I feel I would still have been happy in the knowledge I had done the right thing for both of us, and that the support would have still been there.'

It may be worth asking why women do need 'every little ounce of support and encouragement you can get' to do this very ordinary task. If things have not been easy for you, this book may have helped you to try to make sense of the worries you and others had. The more understanding there is of how breastfeeding works, and how it can be undermined, the more women will be free to choose to do it.

A woman who is capable of making colostrum will make milk. A woman whose milk 'comes in' after birth will not find it 'disappearing' in some unlucky way so that she cannot feed her baby while others can. What makes the difference is simply the ability of the baby to get at the milk she is making. This can be encouraged by improving the way the baby takes a good mouthful of a mother's breast so that she can milk it. Shortening and 'dividing' feeds, and spacing them to suit inaccurate myths about how long babies should go between their feeds will send messages to the body to make less milk, leading to the impression that there is a shortfall, the need for complementary bottles and ultimately the end of breastfeeding. It all seems very simple. But it can be hard to hang on to the true information and disregard the things people say about breastfeeding which are based on their own (or second-hand), experience of it as a vulnerable and difficult process. This is especially hard when you are newly delivered, tired or sore, and a novice at something which seems beyond you. This is partly why women do need help: help to which they and their babies are entitled.

Asking for help

Breastfeeding counsellors do understand how vitally important the smallest concern can feel to a mother who is worried about her baby or about her own capacity to breastfeed. They know she needs someone who will listen uncritically, not contradict her or dismiss those feelings.

---

*'Once it was written into my care plan that
I needed help with breastfeeding, the staff were
all excellent.'*

They know how difficult it can be to ring someone – because it may sound silly, or it may be so important that it is hard to bear the idea that this may be the last chance.

'I knew and liked the breastfeeding counsellor from our NCT class but could not face more advice lest it be different and anyway I could not talk coherently without crying . . . we just wished we'd known then, as we do now, that this is a "normal" reaction to feeding problems.'

'The fact that NCT trains breastfeeding counsellors acknowledges that people do have problems and realises support is vitally important.'

Every mother deserves as much time as it takes to help her to succeed in breastfeeding or to come to terms with not succeeding and should feel she can ask for help until she is satisfied.

Telling the truth

Women have always been grateful for the time spent with them by midwives and health visitors who wanted to help them establish breastfeeding. They have appreciated a kind word, a gentle action, thanking them for time and explanations which gave them confidence in their own capacity to breastfeed. They have often been silent to their helpers about the parts they did not like. For years, women who were asked to fill in charts about feeding their babies which were adapted from the ones used for bottle-feeding have simply lied or made a vague guess about how long the baby was on the breast. In the days when ten minutes was supposed to be the limit, they have written 'ten minutes', when they knew quite well that the truth was that the baby started an hour before. In any case, it seemed a silly question – to many midwives as well – since it was hard to know whether to count all those little pauses. Because of the rules, the feedback for the staff was mostly useless. Perhaps now women are being more honest in their feedback to their helpers in the medical professions and in the voluntary groups, saying what they find helpful and what they find unhelpful.

How could I help?

Having a baby, and some experience of breastfeeding, will have changed you. Once you have had a baby, you see the need to hold open store doors for women with pushchairs. If you are breastfeeding now, you can do a lot to change things, like offering to go into your toddler's nursery school or playgroup to talk about little babies. Taking your baby, you can offer to be 'the mother' for a hospital or NCT class, or to go into school, perhaps with the local NCT group, to talk to the children about this subject.

'The convenience, ease (once established) and everything, has made me feel strongly that people from school age should be encouraged to think positively about it . . .'

You may be the only person to understand the feelings of a breastfeeding mother being asked to leave a restaurant – could you help her ask to stay, or console her if she leaves? Even smiling at a mother who is feeding may help tip the balance for her. 'The more women that are visibly breastfeeding in public the more acceptable it becomes, so long as they are sensitive to other people's feelings.'

If after reading this book your experiences still worry you, consider making sense of them by talking with partners, parents, children – even after several years – or a breastfeeding counsellor, who is experienced in listening carefully.

If breastfeeding was a good experience you may be able to offer hope and point someone to expert help. You can help – even if it did not work for you – by coming to terms with what happened and letting your daughters, sisters, friends, know they have your support in what they hope to do.

Glossary

Areola
The darker circle of skin around the nipple which varies in size and gives the baby a 'target'

Colostrum
Milk produced for the first few days, looking like melted butter and very useful for the baby.

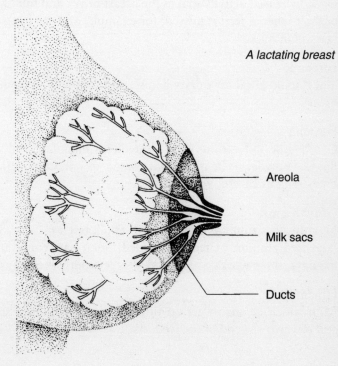

A lactating breast

Areola

Milk sacs

Ducts

Complementary feeds
Feeds given in addition to a breastfeed. These are usually given just after a breastfeed, by bottle or cup. They are usually expected to be of formula, but in some circumstances it is worth considering expressing your own milk to offer.

Demand feeding
A rather unkind way to describe the way in which mothers respond to their baby's realistic needs. 'Responsive' feeding, 'babyled' feeding, and 'flexible' feeding, are all possible alternatives when you are explaining, either to yourself or to others, how the baby is fed, i.e. without timed interference.

Ducts
The tubes leading from the clusters of milk cells to the nipple openings.

Engorgement
Fullness of the breast either at the beginning of breastfeeding when increased activity makes the breast heavy and full of fluid, or later when a feed is missed, for example, and the breasts are just full of milk.

Foremilk
'juicy' milk, good for thirsty babies, and coming first from each breast.

Formula
Cow's milk and various other ingredients manufactured into a fluid or powder to be mixed with water to imitate the effect of breastmilk as carefully as possible.

Growth spurt
Not always a time for extra growth at all, but a period with an increased amount of feeding needed, often happening around ten days, three weeks, six weeks or three months – or any time.

Hindmilk
Milk which begins to get creamy after let-down and creamier still towards the end of the feed.

Inverted nipple
One that turns inwards rather than outwards and so requiring extra care in attaching the baby to the breast.

Let-down
The milk being squeezed down for the baby or tiny muscles in the breast in response to oxytocin. It can happen with no feeling at all, or there can be a warm tingling and gushing, like pins and needles, even occasionally quite painful or pleasurable, and can happen spontaneously.

Mastitis
Inflammation of the breast caused either by an infection or simply milk escaping into the tissue (see page 143).

Milk sacs
Widenings near the end of the ducts carrying milk to the nipple.

'Orthodontic' teat
Claimed by manufacturers to imitate nipples. They may be more acceptable to the breastfed baby.

Oxytocin
Hormone associated with let-down.

Nipple shield
A protective device for the nipple looking like a little Mexican hat in silicone, latex or (if older) rubber. Very old-fashioned ones look like teats on a hard plastic base. These all tend to teach the baby to suck as if bottle-feeding. A shield cuts down the amount of stimulation the baby gives to make more milk.

Prolactin
Hormone all women (and men) have, with increased amounts being secreted after birth, and, especially, in response to breast-feeding, telling the breasts to make more milk.

Thrush (or candida)
A treatable yeast infection which can give mothers sore nipples.

The National Childbirth Trust

You can get information from NCT about breastfeeding counsellors, pump agents, local postnatal groups, etc.:

> The National Childbirth Trust,
> Alexandra House,
> Oldham Terrace,
> Acton,
> LONDON,
> W3 6NH
> Tel: 0181–992 8637

For queries about relactation, feeding adopted babies and use of lactaids, write to Kathy McGlew, c/o NCT (address above), or if you phone, Kathy will get in touch with you.

> Caesarean support (NCT)
> Fiona Barlow
> Tel: 0181-391 1144

The National Childbirth Trust (NCT) is a charity offering information and support in pregnancy, childbirth and early parenthood and aims to enable every parent to make informed choices – including, of course, about breastfeeding.

It is run by, and for, parents through a network of 380 branches and groups throughout Britain (mainly run by volunteers working from home), and offers help and support to members and non-members alike.

Its services range from antenatal classes to postnatal support, and the NCT actively promotes breastfeeding because it believes it offers many advantages to both mother and baby.

Breastfeeding counsellors

There are more than 500 NCT breastfeeding counsellors who have been trained to help mothers establish and continue breastfeeding. They provide information and emotional support to help overcome problems and difficulties, with the aim of enabling mother and baby to breastfeed for as long as they wish.

All NCT teachers and counsellors are highly trained and must re-register every year. Parents are advised to refer any questions about the medical care of mother and baby to their midwife, health visitor or doctor.

The NCT's postnatal support system introduces new mothers and fathers to other parents and children in their area, giving them the opportunity to make new friends and share experiences.

Many NCT mothers and their babies visit primary and secondary schools and colleges to talk about breastfeeding.

A consumer voice

The NCT also provides a consumer voice to ensure that new practices are properly researched, and carries out its own studies among NCT members. This allows the organisation to offer better information to parents and advise health professionals of the feelings and opinions of both expectant couples and parents.

References

p.10
*Howie, *Protective effects of breastfeeding against infection*, <u>British Medical Journal</u>, 1990, 300: 11–16.
Duncan et al, *Exclusive breastfeeding for at least four months protects against Otitis Media*, <u>Pediatrics</u>, 1993, **91: 667–9.
***Byers et al, *Lactation and breast cancer: evidence for a negative association in pre-menopausal women*, <u>American Journal of Epidemiology</u>, 1985, **121**: 664–74; Cumming and Klineberg, <u>International Journal of Epidemiology</u>, 1993, **22**: 684–91.

p.13
*MAIN Trial Collaborative Group, *Preparing for breastfeeding: treatment of inverted and non-protractile nipples in pregnancy*, <u>Midwifery</u>, 1994, **10**: 200–14.

p.23
*Righard and Alade, *Effect of delivery room routines on success of first breast-feed*, <u>The Lancet</u>, 1990, **336**: 1105–07.

p.43
*Goldberg and Adams, *Supplementary water for breast-fed babies in a hot and dry climate – not really a necessity*, <u>Archives of Diseases of Childhood</u>, 1983, **58**: 73–74.

p.57

*deCarvalho et al, *Effects of water supplementation on jaundice in breastfed infants*, <u>Archives of Diseases of Childhood</u>, 1981, 56: 7, pp. 568–69.

p.60

*British Association of Perinatal Medicine et al, *Hypoglycaemia of the newborn: guidelines for appropriate blood glucose screening and treatment of breastfed and bottlefed babies in the UK*, <u>NCT.</u>

p.77

*Whitehead, *Validity of routine clinical test-weighing as a measure of the intake of breastfed babies*, <u>Archives of Diseases of Childhood</u>, 1981, 56: 919–21.

p.85

*Mennello and Beauchamp, <u>The transfer of alcohol to human milk</u>, *New England Journal of Medicine*, 1991, 325:**14**, p. 981–5

p.91

*Chalmers, *Variations in breast feeding and advice, a telephone survey of community midwives and health visitors*, <u>Midwifery</u>, 1991, 7: 162–66.

p.104

*Drewett, Corbett and Wright, *Cognitive and educational attainments of school age children who failed to thrive in infancy: a population study*, <u>Journal of Child Psychology and Psychiatry</u>, 1999, 40, **4**: 551–61.

p.144

*Inch and Fisher, *Mastitis: infection or inflammation?*, <u>The Practitioner,</u> 1995, 239: 572–76.

p.147

*Khin-Maung, *Effect on clinical outcome of breastfeeding during acute diarrhoea*, <u>British Medical Journal</u>, 1985, 290: 587–89.

p.167

*Meir, *Bottle and breastfeeding: effects on transcutaneous oxygen pressure in small preterm infants*, <u>Nursing Research</u>, 1987, **12**:97-105.

Useful reading

Books

Many of the books listed are available from NCT Maternity Sales (address below).

Breastfeeding Your Baby, Moody, Britten and Hogg, NCT Publishing

The Art of Breastfeeding, La Leche League, Angus and Robertson

Successful Breastfeeding, The Royal College of Midwives (written for health professionals, giving up-to-date research behind good practice)

Working Woman's Guide to Breast Feeding, Dana and Price, Meadowbrook Publishing, US (previously *Breastfeeding Guide for the Working Woman*)

Pregnancy and Birth to 5, Health Education Authority (available from your health visitor if you are a first-time mother)

Breastfeeding, Sheila Kitzinger, Dorling Kindersley

The Year After Childbirth, Sheila Kitzinger, Oxford University Press

Bestfeeding, Chloe Fisher, Suzanne Arms and Mary Renfrew, Celestial Arts

Pregnancy, Birth and Parenthood, ed Glynis Tucker, Oxford University Press

The NCT Book of Crying Baby, Anna McGrail, Thorsons/NCT

The NCT Book of Sleep, Penney Hames, Thorsons/NCT

The NCT Book of Safe Foods: What to Eat in Pregnancy, Hannah Hulme Hunter and Rosemary Dodds, Thorsons/NCT (includes eating during breastfeeding)

The NCT Book of First Foods, Ravinder Lilly, Thorsons/NCT

Three in a Bed, Dorothy Jackson, Bloomsbury

When Pregnancy Fails, Borg and Lasker, Routledge and Kegan Paul

Born too Early, Peter Moore, Thorsons

Working Parents' Companion, Teresa Wilson, Thorsons/NCT

Breastfeeding Special Care Babies, Sandra Lang, Bailliere Tindall

NCT leaflets

These are available by post from NCT (Maternity Sales) Ltd, 239 Burnfield Ave, GLASGOW, G46 7TL (Tel: 0141–663 0600, fax: 0141-663 0606, email: sales@nctms.co.uk)

Some of these leaflets are also available on tape – details are on a price list available from the above address.

Leaflets

Breastfeeding – a Good Start (basic information about
  how to begin)
Breastfeeding – Avoiding some of the problems
Breastfeeding – Making Plenty of Milk
Breastfeeding – Too Much Milk
Breastfeeding if Your Baby Needs Special Care
How to Express and Store Breastmilk

Breastfeeding Twins, Triplets or More (Twins & Multiple Birth Association leaflet)
Breastfeeding After a Caesarian Section
Brief Lives – Families Writing about the Death of a Baby

For children

A Hundred and One Things to do with a Baby,
   Jan Ormerod, Viking
Baby Days, Carol Thompson, Orchard
The New Baby, Anne Civardi, Usborne
Welcome to the World, Nickie Siegen-Smith,
   Barefoot Publishing

Useful addresses

If you find difficulty contacting the appropriate organisation, try your local library or information centre for up-to-date contact addresses as the secretaries, addresses and phone numbers of some charities change quite often. The Contact a Family directory (see below) may help.

Many more organisations exist which may help you but space is limited: try a local breastfeeding counsellor and she may be able to put you in touch with one which suits your needs or find an individual from NCT special situations register to speak to.

For babies with special needs

Cleft Lip and Palate Association (CLAPA)
235 Finchley Road
LONDON, NW3 6LS
0171–431 0033
Illustrated leaflet 'Help with feeding', list of special teats, bottles, etc.

BLISS (Baby Life Support Systems)
17–21 Emerald Street
LONDON, WC1 3QL
0171–831 9393

Down's Syndrome Association
155 Mitcham Road
LONDON, SW17 9PG
0181–682 4001

MENCAP
123 Golden Lane
LONDON, EC1Y 0RT
0171–454 0454

Association for Spina Bifida and Hydrocephalus
42 Park Road
PETERBOROUGH, PE1 2UQ
01733–555 099

Contact a Family
170 Tottenham Court Road
LONDON, W1P 0HA
0171–383 3555
Umbrella group for organisations supporting families of
handicapped children. They have a very useful directory *The
CAF directory of specific conditions and rare syndromes in
children with their family support networks.*

For parents who may need extra help

Twins and Multiple Birth Association (TAMBA)
Harnott House
309 Chester Road
Little Sutton
ELLESMERE PORT, CH66 1QQ
Helpline: 0151 348 0020, 7pm–11pm weekdays,
10am–11pm weekends.

Serene (help for parents with crying babies)
B.M. Crysis,
London, WC1N 3XX
0171–404 5011, 8am–11pm 7 days a week

Parents Anonymous, 24 hour tel. Information officer 0171 263 8918

Parentline (incorporating the National Stepfamily Association)
Endway House
The Endway
HADLEIGH
Essex, S57 2AN
01702–559 900

Action for Sick Children (have a leaflet about your rights to stay with your child in hospital)
300 Kingston House
LONDON, SW20 8LX
0181– 542 4848

For mothers

Women's Health
52 Featherstone St.,
LONDON, EC1Y 8RT
0171–251 6580

ParentAbility (organisation for parents with disabilities)
PO Box 72
RUISLIP
Middlesex, HA4 6XU
0160–086 0186

British Diabetic Association,
10 Queen Anne St.,
LONDON, WC1M 0BD
0171–323 1531

Association for Postnatal Illness,
25 Jerdan Place,
Fulham,
LONDON, SW6 1BE
0171–386 0860

The Maternity Alliance
45 Beech Street
LONDON, EC2P 2LX
0171–588 8682

National Council for One-parent Families
225 Kentish Town Road
LONDON, NW5 2LX
0171–428 5400

Meet a Mum Association
26 Avenue Road
South Norwood
LONDON, SE25 4DX
0181–771 5595

Women's Environmental Network
87 Worship Street
LONDON, EC2A 4BE
0171–247 3327

Help with diet

Vegetarian Society
Parkdale,
Dunham Road,
ALTRINCHAM,
Cheshire, WA14 4QG
0161–928 0793

Vegan Society
7 Battle Road
ST LEONARDS ON SEA
East Sussex, TN37 7AA
01424–427 393

If a baby dies

Foundation for the Study of Sudden Infant Death
14 Halkin Street
LONDON, SW1X 7DP
helpline: 0171–235 1721, 24 hours a day

Stillbirth and Neonatal Death Society (SANDS)
28 Portland Place
LONDON, W1N 3DE
0171–436 5881
leaflets: 'Saying goodbye to your baby' and 'Saying hello before you say goodbye'

Compassionate Friends,
53 North Street
BRISTOL, BS3 1EN
0117–953 9639

Other organisations which support breastfeeding mothers

Association of Breastfeeding Mothers
PO Box 207
BRIDGEWATER
Somerset

Breastfeeding Network
PO Box 11126
PAISLEY
Scotland PA2 8YB
0870–900 8787 (to be put in touch with a local supporter)

La Leche League
PO Box 29
West Bridgeford
NOTTINGHAM, NG2 7NP
0171–242 1278

Index

Glossary entries are in **bold**

If you have found this book useful, you may be interested in the following titles published by VERMILION:

You and Your New Baby
by Christine Hill
0 09 181 712 9   £8.99

The Great Ormond Street New Baby and Child Care Book
0 09 185299 4   £14.99

The New Baby and Toddler Sleep Programme
by Dr John Pearce
0 09 182591 1   £7.99

Aromatherapy and Massage for Mother and Baby
by Allison England
0 09 182275 0   £7.99

The Guide to Your Child's Symptoms
edited by Dr David Haslam
0 09 181603 3   £12.99

Twins and Multiple Births
by Dr Carol Cooper
0 09 181471 5   £9.99

Toddler Taming
by Dr Christopher Green
0 09 177258 3   £9.99

To obtain your copy, simply telephone the TBS Direct credit-card
hotline on 01206 255800.